日本医療薬学会
医療薬学用語集

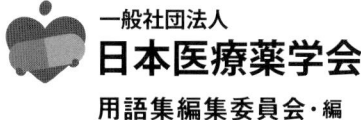
一般社団法人
日本医療薬学会
用語集編集委員会・編

じほう

序　文

　日本医療薬学会の前身である日本病院薬学会は，1990年6月に（社）日本病院薬剤師会が中心となって設立されました．2001年に現在の日本医療薬学会に名称を変更し，2008年12月には一般社団法人となるなど，歴代会頭のリーダーシップのもと着実に学会としての基礎を築き，会員数も9,000人を超えるに至りました．その会員構成は，病院・薬局の薬剤師，薬系大学教員・学生，製薬企業や行政関係者など多岐にわたっています．この四半世紀の間に，医療や教育の世界は大きく変化し，薬剤師が医療の担い手として医療法に明記され，医薬分業が進み，薬剤師の業務が飛躍的に拡大するとともに，薬学教育は6年制に改革されることとなりました．

　医療薬学は，医療の担い手である薬剤師の活動を支える学問的基盤として，基礎薬学から臨床医学まで広範な学問領域と密接に関連するとともに，新しい学問領域を積極的に取り込むことにより，進化・発展を遂げてきました．さらに，clinical pharmacy，pharmaceutical care，collaborative drug therapy managementなど，米国発の新しい概念や行動様式に多大な影響を受けてきました．

　日本医療薬学会の理事会では，医療薬学に関する用語集の刊行について，かねてより議論を重ねてきました．学問研究の進歩が著しい現代において，まだまだ学問としての歴史が浅い医療薬学をしっかり発展させていくためには，用語の整理が不可欠です．学会として新たに英文誌を刊行し，日本発の医療薬学の研究成果をグローバルに発信していくためにも，日本語と英語の双方向の用語の統一を図る必要があります．そこで，設立25周年を迎える本学会の記念事業として用語集刊行を位置付け，アドホックに用語集編集委員会を立ち上げ，金沢大学附属病院教授・薬剤部長の宮本謙一先生に編集委員長をお願いしました．お忙しい中を精力的に用語集の編纂にご尽力いただいた宮本委員長，アドバイザー，編集委員，作業部会，事務局の皆様に，心より感謝申し上げます．

　本用語集は，現在のわが国の医療薬学の到達点を示すとともに，次の四半世紀に向けての出発点となるものです．本書が，医療現場の薬剤師をはじめ，医療薬学に携わる研究者，医療薬学を学ぶ学生諸君など多くの皆様に利用されることにより，医療薬学の新しい展開への礎となることを期待しています．

2014年3月

日本医療薬学会
会頭　安原　眞人

発刊にあたって

　薬剤師の医療への貢献が求められ，臨床の現場で活躍するようになり，薬学教育が6年制となるに至って医療薬学は飛躍的に発展してきました．それに伴って医療薬学関連の学会発表や論文発表も盛んに行われるようになりました．しかし，日本医療薬学会の学術論文誌の英文 Summary や Key Word には怪しげな英語も散見されます．さらに，学会として英文誌の発行も検討されはじめた2012年春，安原会頭から，「医療薬学領域の用語集を取りまとめるように」とのご下命があり，用語集編集委員会で編纂方針を決定後，各領域から協力者を募って作業部会を組織して医療薬学分野で必要と思われる語彙の収集，整理を開始しました．

　本誌の編纂方針の第一は，できる限り医療薬学に必須の用語を収載することでした．したがって，医薬品名，疾病名，病原菌名，汎用でない検査項目や生理・解剖用語は割愛しました．一方，Appendix として，処方に用いられる用語（略語）とアミノ酸の略語表記一覧をのせました．

　方針の第二は，収載数の目標を2,000語とし，日本語－英語－英略語でそれぞれ対訳検索できるものでした．しかし，辞書としての機能は付けず，必要な用語の意味はそれぞれ専門の辞書に当たってもらうことにしました．なお，各用語の訳などを調べた際の参考図書などを巻末に挙げたので，参考にしていただけたら幸いです．

　方針の第三は，2013年度中に編纂を終えてできるだけ早く日本医療薬学会の会員に無料提供することでした．ということで，編集委員や作業部会委員の献身的な努力のおかげで，わずか2年足らずの短期間で出版にこぎつけることができたことを厚く感謝いたします．

　本誌の編纂のなかで最も苦労したのは，この分野には，わが国特有の用語が多いため，適切な英語訳を調べ，選択することでした．したがって，会員はじめ本用語集をご利用の皆様におかれましては，用語の過不足，適切とは思えない用語などお気づきの点が多々あると思いますので，遠慮なくお申し越しいただき，また忌憚のないご意見をお寄せいただいて，本用語集を末永く育てて行っていただきますよう，切にお願い申し上げます．

2014年3月

用語集編集委員会委員長
宮本　謙一

医療薬学用語集執筆者一覧

用語集編集委員会

担当副会頭　鈴木洋史（東京大学医学部附属病院）
委員長　　　宮本謙一（金沢大学医学部附属病院）
委　　員　　望月眞弓（慶應義塾大学薬学部）
　　　　　　山本康次郎（群馬大学医学部附属病院）
アドバイザー　中野眞汎（静岡県立大学客員教授室）
　　　　　　山田勝士（長崎国際大学薬学部）
事務局　　　中澤一純（一般社団法人日本医療薬学会）

作業部会

がん領域　　濱　敏弘（がん研究会有明病院）
　　　　　　篠　道弘（静岡県立静岡がんセンター）
感染領域　　白石　正（山形大学医学部附属病院）
　　　　　　木村利美（東京女子医科大学病院）
統　　計　　奥田千恵子（横浜薬科大学）
医療安全　　岩瀬利康（獨協医科大学病院）
薬　　事　　小野俊介（東京大学薬学部）
製　　剤　　花輪剛久（東京理科大学薬学部）

日本医療薬学会出版委員会

　　　　　　中村敏明（福井大学医学部附属病院）
　　　　　　野田幸裕（名城大学薬学部）

日本医療薬学会編集委員会

　　　　　　賀川義之（静岡県立大学薬学部）
　　　　　　岡村　昇（武庫川女子大学薬学部）

英　名

0-9, α-Ω

1-compartment model　1-コンパートメント・モデル
100% lethal dose　確実致死量　LD_{100}
3-hydroxy-3-methylglutaryl coenzyme A　3-ヒドロキシ-3-メチルグルタリル補酵素A　HMG-CoA
3,4-dihydroxyphenylalanine　3,4-ジヒドロキシフェニルアラニン　DOPA
4M-4E matrix analyzing method　4M-4Eマトリックス分析法
5-hydroxytryptamine (serotonin)　セロトニン　5-HT
5-year observed survival　5年実測生存率
5-year relative survival　5年相対生存率
5-year survival rate　5年生存率
50% effective concentration　50%有効濃度　EC_{50}
50% effective dose　50%有効量　ED_{50}
50% inhibitory concentration　50%阻害濃度　IC_{50}
50% lethal dose　50%致死量　LD_{50}
50% minimum inhibitory concentration　50%最小発育阻止濃度　MIC_{50}
90% minimum inhibitory concentration　90%最小発育阻止濃度　MIC_{90}
α error　α過誤（第一過誤）
α-hemolysis　α-溶血
α-lipoprotein　α-リポタンパク　α-LP
$α_1$-acid glycoprotein　アルファ1-酸性糖タンパク　AGP
β error　β過誤（第二過誤）
β-hemolysis　β-溶血
β-lactamase　β-ラクタマーゼ
γ-aminobutyric acid　γ-アミノ酪酸　GABA
γ-glutamyltranspeptidase　γ-グルタミルトランスペプチダーゼ　γ-GTP

A

ABC analysis　ABC分析，重点分析
abdominal pain　腹痛
abdominal position　腹臥位
abdominal pressure　腹圧
ablactation　離乳
ABO blood group　ABO式血液型
absolute incompatibility　配合不可
absolute risk reduction　絶対リスク減少

absorbance 吸光度
absorption 吸収
absorption rate constant 吸収速度定数 k_a
absorption, distribution, metabolism, and excretion 吸収・分布・代謝・排泄 ADME
absorptive ointment 吸水軟膏 AO
abuse 虐待, 乱用
academic article 学術論文
acceleration test 加速試験
acceptable daily intake 一日許容摂取量 ADI
accessory symptom 随伴症状
accident 事故
acclimation 環境順化
accompanying diseases 副傷病名
accountability 説明責任
acetylcholine アセチルコリン ACh
acetylcholinesterase アセチルコリンエステラーゼ AChE
acid-base balance 酸塩基平衡
acquired immunity 獲得免疫
acquired immunodeficiency syndrome 後天性免疫不全症候群(エイズ) AIDS
acquired resistance 獲得耐性
active controlled study 実薬対照試験
active drug 実薬
active immunity 能動免疫
active ingredient 有効成分
active transport 能動輸送
activities of daily living 日常生活動作 ADL
acute toxicity test 急性毒性試験
addict 常習者
addiction 耽溺, 嗜癖
additive action 相加作用
additives 添加剤
adherence アドヒアランス(患者の治療への積極参加の態度)
adhesiveness 付着性
adipocytokine アディポサイトカイン
adiponectin アディポネクチン
adipose tissue 脂肪組織
adjusted death rate 訂正死亡率
adjuvant chemotherapy 補助化学療法

administrative disposition　行政処分
administrative guidance　行政指導
admission　入院
adrenoceptor（adrenergic receptor）　アドレナリン受容体
adrenocorticotropic hormone　副腎皮質刺激ホルモン　ACTH
adsorbents　吸着剤
adsorption　吸着
adulterated drug　不良医薬品
advance directives　事前指示
advanced cancer　進行癌
advanced cardiovascular life support　二次救命処置　ACLS
advanced medical care　先進医療
advanced treatment hospital　特定機能病院
adverse drug reaction　医薬品有害反応　ADR
adverse drug reaction reporting system　医薬品副作用報告制度
adverse event　有害事象　AE
aerobic infection　好気性感染
aerobic training　有酸素運動
aerosols　エアゾール剤
afferent infectious disease　輸入感染症
afferent nerve　求心性神経
affinity　親和性
afterload　後負荷
agar medium　寒天培地
agarose-gel electrophoresis　アガロースゲル電気泳動　AGE
agate mortar　メノウ乳鉢
agate pestle　メノウ乳棒
age of onset　発症年齢
age pyramid　人口ピラミッド
age-adjusted death rate　年齢調整死亡率
agglutination　凝集反応
aggregation　集合
aging and low birth-rate society　少子高齢化社会
agonist　作動薬
agricultural chemicals　農薬
air pollution　大気汚染
air-borne bacteria　空中浮遊菌
air-borne infection　空気感染

airtight container　気密容器
airway resistance　気道抵抗
alanine aminotransferase　アラニンアミノ基転移酵素　ALT(GPT)
albumin-globulin ratio　アルブミン・グロブリン比　A/G比
alcohol dehydrogenase　アルコール脱水素酵素　ADH
alcohol dependence　アルコール依存症
alcohol-based hand rub　擦式アルコール製剤
aldehyde dehydrogenase　アルデヒド脱水素酵素　ALDH
alkaline phosphatase　アルカリフォスファターゼ　ALP
All Japan Hospital Association　全日本病院協会　AJHA
allergen　アレルゲン(抗原あるいは抗原を含む物質)
allocation　割付
alternative dispute resolution　裁判外紛争解決手続　ADR
alternative medicine　代替医療
ambulance car　救急車
ambulatory care　外来治療
American Association of Pharmaceutical Scientists　米国薬科学会　AAPS
American College of Apothecaries　米国薬局薬剤師会　ACA
American College of Clinical Pharmacy　米国臨床薬学会　ACCP
American Joint Committee on Cancer　対がん米国合同委員会　AJCC
American Pharmacists Association　米国薬剤師会　APhA
American Society of Clinical Oncology　米国臨床腫瘍学会　ASCO
American Society of Health-System Pharmacists　米国医療薬剤師会(病院薬剤師会に相当)　ASHP
amorphous　無晶形(非晶質)
amphoteric surface active agents　両性界面活性剤
ampule　アンプル　A
anaerobic culture　嫌気培養
anaerobic infection　嫌気性感染症
analysis of variance　分散分析　ANOVA
anamnese　アナムネ(初診時の問診)(独)
anaphylaxis　アナフィラキシー
anatomical therapeutic chemical classification system　ATC分類(解剖治療化学分類法)　ATC
androgen receptor　アンドロゲン受容体　AR
angiogenesis　血管新生
angiography　血管造影
angiotensin converting enzyme　アンジオテンシン変換酵素　ACE

angle of repose　安息角
anion gap　陰イオンギャップ
anionic surface active agents　陰イオン界面活性剤
Annual Health, Labour and Welfare Report　厚生労働白書
anonymizing　匿名化
antacids　制酸薬
antagonism　拮抗
antagonist　拮抗薬
antedrug　アンテドラッグ（局所で作用して吸収後，不活性となる薬）
antidiarrheal drugs　止瀉薬
anti-doping　反ドーピング
anti-inflammatory drugs　抗炎症薬
antibacterial agents　抗菌薬
antibacterial spectrum　抗菌スペクトル
antibiotic resistance　抗生物質耐性
antibiotics　抗生物質
antibody　抗体　Ab
antibody-dependent cellular cytotoxicity　抗体依存性細胞障害　ADCC
anticancer drugs　抗がん薬
anticarcinogen　発がん抑制物質
anticoagulants　抗凝固薬
antidiuretic hormone　抗利尿ホルモン（バソプレシン）　ADH
antidote　解毒薬
antiemetics　制吐薬
antifungal agents　抗真菌薬
antifungal spectrum　抗真菌スペクトラム
antifungal（antimycotic）activity　抗真菌作用
antigen　抗原　Ag
antigen presentation cell　抗原提示細胞　APC
antigen-binding fragment　抗原結合性フラグメント　Fab
antimicrobial use density　抗菌薬使用密度　AUD
antinuclear antibodies　抗核抗体　ANA
antioxidants　抗酸化剤
antipseudomonal agents　抗緑膿菌薬
antipyretic analgesics　解熱鎮痛薬
antiseptic hand rub　擦式手指消毒
antiseptic handwash　手洗い消毒
antituberculous agents　抗結核薬

antitussives　鎮咳薬
antiviral agents　抗ウイルス薬
aphthous stomatitis　アフタ性口内炎
apoenzyme　アポ酵素
apoprotein　アポタンパク質
apoptosis　アポトーシス
apothanasia　延命(延命治療)
apparent infection　顕性感染
application for the manufacture and sales approval　製造販売承認申請
application of approval　承認申請
appropriate use of drug　(医薬品の)適正使用
Approved Drug Products with Therapeutic Equivalence Evaluations　オレンジブック(米国)
area under the blood concentration vs. time curve　血中濃度-時間曲線下面積　AUC
aromatic amino acid　芳香族アミノ酸　AAA
arterial CO_2 pressure　動脈血二酸化炭素分圧　Pa_{CO_2}
arterial O_2 pressure　動脈血酸素分圧　Pa_{O_2}
arterial O_2 saturation　動脈血酸素飽和度　Sa_{O_2}
Arthus's reaction　アルサス反応(Ⅲ型アレルギー反応の一種)
artificial saliva　人工唾液
ascending infection　上行性感染
asepsis　無菌
aspartate aminotransferase　アスパラギン酸-アミノ基転移酵素　AST(GOT)
aspiration pneumonia　誤嚥性肺炎
aspirin-induced asthma　アスピリン喘息
assent　同意
assessment　評価
Association of International Foods and Nutrition　国際栄養食品協会　AIFN
atomic absorption spectrophotometry　原子吸光光度法
ATP-binding cassette transporter(ABC transporter)　ABC輸送担体
atrial natriuretic peptide　心房性ナトリウム利尿ペプチド　ANP
atrioventricular block　房室ブロック(AVブロック)
attending physician　主治医
attenuated vaccine　弱毒化ワクチン
audit　監査
auditor　監査担当者
autoclave　高圧蒸気滅菌器
autologous bone marrow transplantation　自家骨髄移植

automated external defibrillator　自動体外式除細動器　AED
automated peritoneal dialysis　自動腹膜透析　APD
autonomic nerve　自律神経
autopsy　剖検
autotransfusion　自己血輸血
average drug concentration at steady state　定常状態平均薬物濃度　$C_{ss\,av}$
average number of hospitalization　平均在院日数
avian influenza　鳥インフルエンザ
avirulence　非病原性

B

Bacille de Calmette et Guerin（仏）　BCGワクチン　BCG
background　背景
bactereriolysis　溶菌
bacterial contamination　細菌汚染
bacterial eradication rate　除菌率
bacterial examination test　細菌学的検査
bacterial food poisoning　細菌性食中毒
bacterial spore　胞子(芽胞)
bacterial toxin　細菌毒素
bacteriocidal action　殺菌作用
bacteriostatic action　静菌作用
barcode system　バーコードシステム
barrier equipment　防護製品
basal body temperature　基礎体温　BBT
basal energy expenditure　基礎エネルギー消費量　BEE
basal metabolic rate　基礎代謝率　BMR
base　基剤
basic life support　一次救命処置　BLS
Bayesian method（Bayesian inference）　ベイジアン法(ベイズ推計)
bed control　病床管理
behabioral therapy　行動療法
benign　良性の
best-in-class　画期的新薬(ピカ新)
best supportive care　症状に合わせたケア(治療)をすること
bi-levels of positive airway pressures　二相性気道腸圧　BiPAP
bias　バイアス(偏り)

biliary drainage　胆道ドレナージ
biliary excretion　胆汁排泄
binary variable　2値変数
bio-safety level　感染性因子に対する安全性の格付け（生物学的危険度レベル）　BSL
bio-similar　バイオ後続品
bioavailability　生物学的利用能
biochemical modulation　生化学的効果修飾
biochemical oxygen demand　生物化学的酸素要求量　BOD
bioequivalence　生物学的同等性　BE
bioethics　生命倫理
biofilm　バイオフィルム
biohazard　バイオハザード
biological clean room　バイオクリーンルーム
biological containment　生物学的封じ込め
biological false positive　生物学的偽陽性　BFP
biological half-life　生物学的半減期
biological products　生物由来製品
biomarker　生物学的指標
biotechnology　バイオテクノロジー
biotechnology product　組み換え医薬品
bitter stomachic　苦味健胃薬
black box warning　添付文書上の警告（米国）
bleeding tendency　出血傾向
bleeding time　出血時間
blind review　盲検下レビュー
blinding　盲検化
blood coagulation factor　血液凝固因子
blood culture　血液培養
blood flow limited　血流律速
blood flow rate　血流量
blood gas analysis　血液ガス分析
blood glucose　血糖
blood pressure　血圧
blood urea nitrogen　血中尿素窒素　BUN
blood vessel　血管
blood-brain barrier　血液脳関門　BBB
blood-placental barrier　血液胎盤関門
blue letter　安全性速報

Board Certified HIV Pharmacy Specialist　HIV感染症専門薬剤師（日本病院薬剤師会）　BCHIVPS
Board Certified Clinical Pharmacist, Japanese Society of Clinical Pharmacology and Therapeutics　認定薬剤師（日本臨床薬理学会）
Board Certified Clinical Research Coodinator, Japanese Society of Clinical Pharmacology and Therapeutics　認定CRC（日本臨床薬理学会）
Board Certified Infection Control Pharmacy Specialist　感染制御専門薬剤師（日本病院薬剤師会）　BCICPS
Board Certified Oncology Pharmacy Specialist　がん専門薬剤師（日本病院薬剤師会）　BCOPS
Board Certified Pharmacist in Infection Control　感染制御認定薬剤師（日本病院薬剤師会）　BCPIC
Board Certified Pharmacist in Oncology Pharmacy　がん薬物療法認定薬剤師（日本病院薬剤師会）　BCPOP
Board Certified Pharmacist in Pharmacotherapy during Pregnancy and Lactation　妊婦・授乳婦薬物療法認定薬剤師（日本病院薬剤師会）　BCPPPL
Board Certified Pharmacist in Psychiatric Pharmacy　精神科薬物療法認定薬剤師（日本病院薬剤師会）　BCPPP
Board Certified Pharmacy Specialist in Pharmacotherapy during Pregnancy and Lactation　妊婦・授乳婦専門薬剤師（日本病院薬剤師会）　BCPSPPL
Board Certified Psychiatric Pharmacy Specialist　精神科専門薬剤師（日本病院薬剤師会）　BCPPS
Board Certified Tutorial Clinical Pharmacist, Japanese Society of Clinical Pharmacology and Therapeutics　指導薬剤師（日本臨床薬理学会）
body fat percentage　体脂肪率　BFP
body mass index　体格指数　BMI
body surfase area　体表面積　BSA
bone density　骨密度
bone marrow transplantation　骨髄移植　BMT
bone mineral density　骨塩密度　BMD
bone morphogenetic protein　骨形成誘導タンパク　BMP
bone resorption　骨吸収
Bonferroni correction　ボンフェローニの補正
boron delivery system　ホウ素薬剤送達システム　BDS
boron neutron capture therapy　ホウ素中性子捕捉療法　BNCT
bovine serum albumin　ウシ血清アルブミン　BSA
bovine spongiform encephalopathy　ウシ海綿状脳症　BSE
bowel movement　排便

bowel sound 腸雑音
box and whisker plot 箱ひげ図
brain cerebrospinal fluid barrier 脳脊髄液関門 BCSFB
brain death 脳死
branched-chain amino acid and tyrosine molar ratio 総分岐鎖アミノ酸/チロシンモル比 BTR
branched-chain amino acids 分枝鎖アミノ酸 BCAA
brand-name drug 先発医薬品
breath sound 呼吸音 BS
bridging study ブリッジング試験
bringing medicine 持参薬
bronchoalveolar lavage 気管支肺胞洗浄 BAL
bronchodilator 気管支拡張薬
bronchofiberscopy 気管支ファイバースコープ BF
broth dilution method 液体希釈法
broth microdilution method 微量液体希釈法
buccal tablet バッカル錠(口腔剤)
buffer agents 緩衝剤
bulk drug substance 原薬
burden of proof 立証責任

C

C-reactive protein C反応性タンパク CRP
cabinet order 政令
calibration curve 検量線
cancellation of approval 承認の取り消し
Cancer Control Law がん対策基本法
cancer registration がん登録
Cannabis Control Law 大麻取締法
capillary electrophoresis キャピラリー電気泳動
capsules カプセル剤
carcinoembryonic antigen 癌胎児性抗原 CEA
carcinogen 発がん物質
carcinogenesis がん化
carcinogenic test 発がん性試験
carcinogenicity 発がん性
carcinoma 癌腫

carcinomatous pain, cancer pain がん性疼痛
cardiac index 心係数　CI
cardiac output 心拍出量
cardioangiography 心血管造影　CAG
cardiopulmonary arrest 心肺停止　CPA
cardiopulmonary bypass 人工心肺　CPB
cardiopulmonary resuscitation 心肺蘇生　CPR
cardiothoracic ratio 心胸郭比　CTR
care 介護
care manager(long-term care support specialist) ケアマネジャー(介護支援専門員)
carried over effect 持ち越し効果
carrier-mediated transport 担体輸送
case conference 症例検討会
case report form 症例報告書　CRF
case-control study 患者対照研究
catabolism 異化
cataplasms パップ剤
catchment area 診療圏
catechol-O-methyltransferase カテコール-O-メチル基転移酵素　COMT
catheter infection カテーテル感染
causal relationship 因果関係
causative organism 原因菌
cell culture 細胞培養
cell cycle 細胞周期
cell division 細胞分裂
Centers for Disease Control and Prevention 米国疾病予防管理センター　CDC
central nervous system 中枢神経系　CNS
Central Social Insurance Medical Council 中央社会保険医療協議会(中医協)
cerebrospinal fluid 脳脊髄液　CSF
certificate of narcotics receipt 麻薬譲受証
certificate of narcotics transfer 麻薬譲渡証
certified nurse specialist 専門看護師　CNS
certified physician or surgeon 認定医
chemical equilibrium 化学平衡
chemical equivalents 化学的同等製剤
chemical mediator 化学伝達物質
chemical oxygen demand 化学的酸素要求量　COD
chemoembolization 化学塞栓療法

chemoprophylaxis　予防的化学療法
chemoradiotherapy　化学放射線療法
chemoreceptor trigger zone　化学受容器引金帯　CTZ
chemotherapeutic agent　化学療法薬
chemotherapy　化学療法
chewable tablet　チュアブル錠（咀嚼錠）
Cheyne-Stokes breathing　チェーン・ストークス呼吸　CSB
chi-square test　X（カイ）2乗検定
chief complaint　主訴
child-resistant packaging　対小児安全包装　CRP
chimeric antibody　キメラ抗体
chimeric gene　キメラ遺伝子
Chinese herbal medicine　漢方薬
Chinese Pharmaceutical Association　中国薬学会　CPA
chirality　不斉（対掌性）
cholesteryl ester transfer protein　コレステリルエステル転送タンパク　CETP
cholinesterase　コリンエステラーゼ　ChE
chromosome　染色体
chronic obstructive pulmonary disease　慢性閉塞性肺疾患　COPD
chronic toxicity test　慢性毒性試験
chronopharmacology　時間薬理学
chronotherapy　時間治療
chronotropic action　変時作用
circadian rhythm　日内変動
civil liability　民事責任
clean bench　クリーンベンチ
clearance　クリアランス　CL
clinic with beds for inpatients　有床診療所
clinic-pathological conference　臨床病理検討会
clinical audit　診療評価
clinical dose　臨床用量
clinical epidemiology　臨床疫学
clinical equivalence　臨床的同等性
clinical finding　臨床所見
clinical history　病歴
clinical indicator　臨床指標
clinical investigator　治験担当医師
clinical outcome evaluation　診療アウトカム評価

clinical pathway　クリニカルパス
clinical pharmaceutics　臨床薬剤学
clinical pharmacokinetics　臨床薬物動態学
clinical pharmacology　臨床薬理学
clinical pharmacy　臨床薬学
clinical pharmacy practice　臨床薬学的業務
clinical practice　臨床診療，臨床研修
clinical practice guideline　診療ガイドライン
clinical psychologist　臨床心理士
clinical record　臨床記録
clinical research　臨床研究
clinical research associate　治験モニタリング担当者（モニター）　CRA
clinical research coordinator　治験コーディネーター　CRC
clinical results　臨床成績
clinical stage　臨床進行度
clinical study　臨床試験
clinical test　臨床検査
clinical trial　治験　CT
clinical trial administration office　治験事務局
clinics　診療所
clouding of consciousness　意識混濁
cluster analysis, clustering　クラスタ分析
coating agents　コーティング剤
code of ethics　倫理綱領
Code of Ethics for Pharmacist　薬剤師倫理規定
coding region　翻訳領域
coefficient of variation　変動係数　CV
cohort study　コホート研究
cold application　冷罨法
cold sterilization　低温滅菌
collaborative drug therapy management　共同薬物治療管理業務　CDTM
collaborative pharmacy practice　協働薬物治療の実践（プライマリ・ケアにおける医師と薬剤師の連携）　CPP
colloid osmotic pressure　膠質浸透圧
colony forming unit　コロニー形成単位　CFU
colony stimulating factor　コロニー刺激因子　CSF
combination chemotherapy　併用化学療法
combination drugs　配合剤

combination therapy 併用療法
combined effect 併用効果
combined vaccine 混合ワクチン
commission error コミッションエラー(やり損ない)
common drugs 普通薬
Common Technical Document 日米EU3極共通の医薬品承認申請様式 CTD
Common Terminology Criteria for Adverse Event 有害事象共通用語規準 CTCAE
communication skill コミュニケーション能力
community acquired infection 市中感染
community acquired pneumonia 市中肺炎
community pharmacy 市中薬局(地域薬局)
comorbidity 併発症
comparable drug 同種同効薬
comparative negligence 過失相殺
comparison between groups 群間比較
compassionate use (未承認薬の)人道的使用 CU
compatibility 配合変化
compensation for damages 損害賠償
compensation for health damage 健康被害補償
competence 適格性(包括的な臨床能力)
competitive antagonism 競合的拮抗
competitive inhibition 競合的阻害
complaint management 苦情処理
complementary DNA 相補的DNA cDNA
complementary medicine 補完医療
complete response 完全寛解 CR
complexation 複合体形成
compliance 法令順守
complication 合併症
comprehensive medical care 包括医療
computed(computerized) tomography コンピュータ断層撮影 CT
computer based test 知識および問題解決能力を評価するコンピュータを用いた客観試験 CBT
concomitant drug 併用薬
confidence interval 信頼区間 CI
confidentiality 守秘義務
confirmatory study 検証的試験
conflict of interest 利益相反 COI

conformity 適合
confounding factor 交絡因子
conjugation 抱合反応
consciousness of disease 病識
conservative therapy 保存療法
consolidation therapy 強化療法(地固め療法)
constipation 便秘
consultation 対診
contact inhibition 接触阻害
content uniformity test 含量均一性試験
content validity 内的妥当性
continuous administration 持続投与
continuous ambulatory peritoneal dialysis 連続携行式腹膜透析　CAPD
continuous hemodiafiltration 持続的血液濾過透析　CHDF
continuous intravenous infusion 持続点滴静注
continuous quality improvement 継続的質改善　CQI
continuous variable 連続変数
contiuous subcutaneous insulin infusion 持続皮下インスリン注入療法　CSII
contraception 避妊
contract research organization 医薬品開発業務受託機関　CRO
contraindication 禁忌
control drug 対照薬
control group 対照群
controlled clinical trial 比較臨床試験
controlled release 放出制御　CR
controller コントローラー(割り付け担当者)
conventional animal 普通動物
cooperation clinical pathway 地域連携クリニカルパス
coordinating committee 治験調整委員会
coordinating investigator 治験調整医師
coronary artery bypass 冠動脈バイパス(A-Cバイパス)
coronary care unit 冠動脈疾患集中治療室(内科系集中治療室)　CCU
correlation coefficient 相関係数　r
corticotropin 副腎皮質刺激ホルモン　ACTH
corticotropin releasing hormone 副腎皮質刺激ホルモン放出ホルモン　CRH
cosmetics 化粧品
cosolvate 溶媒和
cost management 原価管理

cost-benefit　費用対効果
counseling　心理療法(カウンセリング)
counterfeit drug　にせ薬
course　コース(クール)
covariate　共変量
cox proportional hazard regression analysis　コックス比例ハザード回帰分析
creatine kinase　クレアチン・キナーゼ　CK
creatinine clearance　クレアチニン・クリアランス　CL_{cr}, C_{cr}
criminal liability　刑事責任
crisis management　危機管理
critical appraisal　批判的吟味
critical relative humidity　臨界相対湿度　CRH
cross infection　交差感染
cross reaction　交差反応
cross resistance　交差耐性
cross-sectional study　横断研究
crossover trial　交差試験
crystalline polymorphism　結晶多形
crystallization　結晶化
cumulative effect　蓄積効果
curative treatment　根治的治療
curriculum vitae　履歴書　CV
customer satisfaction analysis　顧客満足度分析　CS分析
cyclooxygenase　シクロオキシゲナーゼ　COX
cytochrome P450　チトクロム P450　CYP
cytodiagnosis　細胞診
cytokine　サイトカイン
cytotoxicity　細胞毒性
cytotoxin　細胞毒

D

daily dose　一日投与量
data and safety monitoring board　効果・安全性評価委員会
date of admission　入院日
date of manufacture　製造年月日
day care　デイ・ケア
day surgery　日帰り手術

de novo pathway 新生経路
de novo synthesis 新規生合成
dead on arrival 到着時死亡　DOA
death conference 死亡症例検討会
death from overwork 過労死
death with dignity 尊厳死
declaration of Geneva ジュネーブ宣言
declaration of Helsinki ヘルシンキ宣言
decoctions 煎剤
deep burn Ⅲ度熱傷
deep dermal burn 深達性Ⅱ度熱傷
deep vein thrombosis 深在静脈血栓症　DVT
defective drug 欠陥医薬品
definite diagnosis 確定診断
definitive radiation therapy 根治的放射線治療
deglutition 嚥下
degree of freedom 自由度　df
dehydration 脱水
delayed hypersensitivity 遅延性過敏症
delayed type allergy 遅延型アレルギー
deleterious substance 劇物
Deming's cycle デミングサイクル（PDCAサイクル）
dendritic cell 樹状細胞　DC
dentist 歯科医師
deoxyribonucleic acid デオキシリボ核酸　DNA
dependence test 依存性試験
dependency 依存
dependent drug 依存性薬物
dependent variable 従属変数
desensitization therapy 減感作療法
DESIGN 褥瘡状態評価法（depth, exudate, size, inflammation/ infection, granulation, necrotic tissue）
designated cancer care hospital がん診療連携拠点病院
designated communicable disease 指定伝染病
designated disease 特定疾患
designated drug 指定医薬品
designated infection disease control hospital 感染症指定医療機関
detection limit 検出限界

detergents　洗浄剤
detoxication　解毒
diabetes mellitus　糖尿病　DM
diagnosis　診断　Dx
diagnosis procedure combination　診断群分類(包括医療評価制度における)　DPC
diagnosis related group/prospective payment system　診断群別包括支払方式　DRG/PPS
diagnostic and statistical manual of mental disorders　精神障害の診断と統計の手引き　DSM
diagnostic drug　診断薬
diagnostic support system　診断支援システム
dialysis　透析
diarrhea　下痢
diet therapy　食事療法
dietary supplement　健康食品(サプリメント)
diffusion　拡散
diluents　希釈剤，賦形剤
dipeptidyl peptidase 4　インクレチンの不活性化酵素　DPP-4
diphtheria-pertussis-tetanus vaccine　三種(ジフテリア・百日咳・破傷風)混合ワクチン　DPTワクチン
direct access　直接閲覧
direct hemoperfusion　直接血液吸着療法　DHP
direct-to-consumer　医療用医薬品の一般大衆への情報提供のこと　DTC
disappearance rate　消失率
disaster medical assistance team　災害派遣医療チーム　DMAT
disaster medical center　災害拠点病院
disaster medicine　災害医療
discharge summary　退院要約(退院時サマリー)
disclosure of medical records　診療録の開示
disclosure of patient information　診療情報開示
discontinuation criteria　中止基準
discrete variable　離散変数
disease free survival　無病生存期間　DFS
disease notification　告知
disease staging　病期分類
disease-modifying antirheumatic drugs　疾患修飾性抗リウマチ薬　DMARDs
disinfection　消毒
disintegration test　崩壊試験法

Dispense As Written　後発品変更不可処方せん（米）　DAW
dispense by counting　計数調剤
dispense by weight or volumetric　計量調剤
dispensing　調剤
dispensing error　調剤ミス
dispensing fee　調剤技術料，調剤報酬
dispensing record　調剤録
dispersion　ばらつき
disposables　ディスポーザブル製剤
disseminated intravascular coagulation　播種性血管内凝固症候群　DIC
dissociation constant　解離定数
dissolution　溶解
dissolution test　溶出試験
distilled water　蒸留水　DW
distribution　分布
distribution volume　分布容積　Vd
ditto prescription　Do処方（前回処方と同じ内容を繰り返して処方すること）
dizziness　めまい
doctor letter　緊急安全性情報（イエローペーパー）
documentation　文書化
domestic violence　家庭内暴力（ドメスティック・バイオレンス）　DV
dosage　薬用量，放射線量
dosage and administration　用法用量
dosage design　投与設計
dosage form　投与剤形
dosage regimen　投与計画
dose limiting factor　用量規制因子　DLF
dose limiting toxicity　用量制限毒性　DLT
dose of radiation　照射線量
dose response relationship　用量相関
dose response study　用量反応試験
dose-finding study　用量設定試験
dosing period　投与期間
double blind controlled trial　二重盲検比較試験
double blind test　二重盲検試験　DBT
double dummy　ダブルダミー
drip infusion　点滴　DI
drip rate　滴下速度

droplet infection　飛沫感染
drug abuse　薬物乱用
drug allergy　薬物アレルギー
drug concentration at steady state　定常状態　C_{ss}
drug delivery system　薬物送達システム　DDS
drug dependence　薬物依存
drug development　創薬
drug event monitoring　薬剤イベントモニタリング　DEM
drug information　医薬品情報　DI
drug lag　ドラッグ・ラグ（医薬品承認審査遅滞）
drug management　医薬品管理
drug master file　原薬等登録原簿　DMF
drug packing paper〔medicine wrapping paper, charta（ラテン）〕　薬包紙
drug price in National Health Insurance scheme　薬価
Drug Price List　薬価基準
drug pricing system based on brand　銘柄別収載方式
drug profile book　お薬手帳
drug re-evaluation system　医薬品再評価制度
drug re-examination system　医薬品再審査制度
drug rearing　育薬
drug resistance　薬剤耐性
drug rush　薬疹
Drug Safety Update　医薬品安全対策情報　DSU
drug substitution　代替調剤
drug susceptibility test　薬剤感受性試験
drug transporter　薬物輸送担体
drug-drug interaction　薬物間相互作用
drug-eluting stent　薬剤溶出ステント
Pharmaceutical Affairs Law　薬事法　PAL
drugs classified as record keeping items　記帳義務医薬品
drugs not in the Japanese Pharmacopoeia　日本薬局方外医薬品
dry air sterilization　乾熱滅菌
dry powder inhaler　粉末製剤吸入器　DPI
dry syrup　ドライシロップ　DS
dual energy x-ray absorptiometry　二重エネルギーX線吸収測定法　DEXA法
Dunnett's test　ダネットの検定

E

ear drops　点耳剤
early exposure　早期臨床体験学習
early postmarketing phase vigilance　市販直後調査　EPPV
echography　超音波診断
economy-class syndrome　静脈血栓塞栓症（エコノミークラス症候群）
effective concentration　有効濃度　EC
efferent nerve　遠心性神経
effervescent tablet　発泡錠
efficiency half life　有効半減期
efflux　排出
ejection fraction　駆出率　EF
electrocardiogram　心電図　ECG
electrochemical detector　電気化学検出器　ECD
electroencephalogram　脳波　EEG
electromyogram　筋電図　EMG
electron spin resonance　電子スピン共鳴　ESR
electronic data capture　電子データ収集　EDC
electronic medical record　電子診療録　EMR
electrophoresis　電気泳動
elemental diet　成分栄養　ED
eligible patient　適格患者
elimination half-life　消失半減期　$t_{1/2}$
elimination rate constant　消失速度定数　k_e
elixirs　エリキシル剤
embryonic stem cell　ES 細胞，胚性幹細胞　ES cell
emergency and critical care center　救命救急センター
emergency contraceptive　緊急避妊薬　EC
emergency medical technician　救急救命士
emergency room　救急治療室　ER
emerging infectious disease　新興感染症
emetics　催吐薬
empathic attitude　共感的態度
empiric therapy　経験的治療
emulsifiers　乳化剤
emulsions　乳剤
enantiomer　鏡像異性体

endemic disease　風土病
endocytosis　エンドサイトシス（細胞の食作用，飲作用）
endoscopic operation(surgery)　内視鏡下手術
endotoxin　内毒素
endpoint　評価項目
enemas　浣腸
enteral nutrition　経腸栄養法　EN
enteric coated tablet　腸溶錠
enterohepatic circulation　腸肝循環
envelope for drugs　薬袋
environmental hormones　環境ホルモン
environmental impact assessment　環境アセスメント（環境影響評価）　EIA
environmental pollution　環境汚染
enzyme immunoassay　酵素免疫測定法　EIA
enzyme-linked immunosorbent assay　エライザ法，酵素結合免疫測定法　ELISA
epidemiology　疫学
epidermal burn　Ⅰ度熱傷　EB
epidermal growth factor　上皮細胞増殖因子　EGF
epitope　抗原決定基
equity　公正性
equivalence trial　同等性試験
error proof　エラーの発生や波及の防止
erythrocyte sedimentation rate　赤血球沈降速度　ESR
essential amino acid　必須アミノ酸　EAA
essential amino acids/non-essential amino acids ratio　必須アミノ酸/非必須アミノ酸比　E/N比
essential document　必須文書
essential drug　必須医薬品　E-drug
essential fatty acid　必須脂肪酸　EFA
esterified cholesterol to total cholesterol ratio　コレステロールエステル/総コレステロール比　EC/TC
estimated glomerular filtration rate　推算糸球体濾過量　eGFR
ethical drug　医療用医薬品
ethical guidelines for epidemiological research　疫学研究の倫理指針
ethics code in medicine　医の倫理綱領
ethics committee　倫理委員会
ethnic differences　人種差
eutectic point　共融点

evidence-based medicine　科学的根拠に基づく医療　EBM
excipients　添加剤
exclusion criteria　除外基準
excretion　排泄
exercise therapy　運動療法
exocytosis　エクソサイトシス(細胞の開口分泌，開口放出)
expectorants　去痰薬
expensive medical charge　高額療養費
expensive medical charge insurance　高額療養費支給制度
expert evidence　鑑定(鑑定書)
expiration date　使用期限
explaining treatment plan on discharge　退院時療養計画書
exploratory data analysis　探索的データ解析　EDA
exploratory study　探索的試験
extensive metabolizer　高代謝能保持者　EM
external exposure　体外被曝
external medicine　外用薬
extracellular fluid　細胞外液
extraction ratio　除去率，抽出率
extracts　エキス剤
extramural dispensing　院外調剤

F

face pain rating scale　疼痛表情評価スケール
facilitated diffusion　促進拡散
faculty development　大学教員資質開発　FD
failsafe　二重安全装置
fair competition code　公正競争規約
Fair Trade Conference　公正取引協議会
family history　家族歴
fasting blood sugar　空腹時血糖　FBS
fatality rate　致死率
feasibility study　実行可能性調査
Federation of Asian Pharmaceutical Association　アジア薬剤師連盟　FAPA
fee schedule for dispensing　調剤報酬点数表
fee schedule for medical services　診療報酬点数表
fee-for-service system　出来高払い制度

feto-maternal infection　母子感染
film-coated tablet　フィルムコーティング錠
filtration fraction　ろ過率　FF
filtration sterilization　ろ過滅菌
fine granules　細粒剤
finger tip unit　塗布量の単位　FTU
first medical interview　初診時の問診（アナムネ）
first pass effect　初回通過効果
first-in-man(human) study　ヒト初回投与試験　FIM
first-order absorption　一次吸収
first-order elimination　一次消失
Fischer ratio　フィッシャー比（分岐鎖アミノ酸（BCAA）と芳香族アミノ酸（AAA）のモル比）
Fisher's exact test　フィッシャーの直接確率検定
five right(drug, dose, route, time, patient)　5つのR（医療事故防止標語）　5R
flavoring substance　矯味剤
flora　常在菌
flow-limited drug　血流速度依存型薬物
fluid extracts　流エキス剤
folk medicine　民間薬（民間療法）
Food and Drug Administration　米国食品医薬品局　FDA
food for specified health uses　特定保健用食品
food poisoning　食中毒
food with health claims　保健機能食品
food with nutrient function claims　栄養機能食品
fool-proof　フールプルーフ（エラーの未然防止）
forced expiratory volume in 1 sec　呼吸1秒量　FEV_1
foreign insoluble matter test for injections　不溶性異物検査法
formative evaluation　形成的評価
formulation　製剤
Fourier transform　フーリエ変換　FT
fractional inhibitory concentration index　薬理学的協力作用を表す指標　FIC index
Franz's cell　フランツセル（膜透過試験システム）
free drug　遊離型薬物（非結合型薬物）
Freedom Of Information　情報開示　FOI
freezing point depression method　氷点降下度法
French-American-British classification　急性白血病のフランス-アメリカ-イギリス分類

FAB 分類
fresh frozen plasma 新鮮凍結血漿　FFP
friability test 摩損度試験
full analysis set 最大の解析対象集団　FAS
functional independence measure 機能的自立度評価法

G

gargles 含嗽剤
gas chromatography-mass spectrometry ガスクロマトグラフ質量分析　GC-MS
gastric emptying rate 胃排出速度　GER
gastric emtying time 胃内容排出時間　GET
gastrointestinal 胃腸の(消化管の)　GI
gelation ゲル化
gender differences 性差
gene library 遺伝子ライブラリー
gene manipulation 遺伝子操作
gene mutation 遺伝子突然変異
gene polymorphism 遺伝子多型
gene recombination 遺伝子組み換え
gene therapy 遺伝子治療
general medical examination 一般健康診断
general physician 総合医
general practitioner 一般開業医　GP
generic drug ジェネリック医薬品，後発医薬品　GE
generic name prescription 一般名処方
generic substitution 後発医薬品への代替調剤
genetic counseling 遺伝カウンセリング(遺伝相談)
genetic diagnosis 遺伝子診断
genomics 遺伝学(ゲノム解析)
genotype 遺伝子型
geriatric health care facility 老人保健施設
geriatric hospital 老人病院
glomerular filtration rate 糸球体濾過速度　GFR
glucagon-like peptide-1 グルカゴン様ペプチド-1　GLP-1
gluconeogenesis 糖新生
glucose challenge test ブドウ糖チャレンジ試験　GCT
glucose tolerance test ブドウ糖負荷試験，耐糖能試験　GTT

glucose transporter　グルコース輸送担体　GLUT
glucose-dependent insulinotropic polypeptide　十二指腸から分泌されるインスリン分泌性ホルモン　GIP
glutamic oxaloacetic transaminase　グルタミン酸オキザロ酢酸トランスアミラーゼ　GOT(AST)
glutamic pyruvic transaminase　グルタミン酸ピルビン酸トランスアミナーゼ　GPT(ALT)
glycolysis　解糖
Good Clinical Practice　医薬品の臨床試験の実施の基準　GCP
Good Industrial Large Scale Practice　優良工業製造規範　GILSP
Good Laboratory Practice　医薬品の安全性に関する非臨床試験の実施の基準　GLP
Good Manufacturing Practice　医薬品及び医薬部外品の製造管理及び品質管理の基準　GMP
Good Pharmacy Education Practice　薬学教育に関する規範　GPEP
Good Pharmacy Practice　薬局業務規範　GPP
Good Postmarketing Study Practice　医薬品の製造販売後調査の実施の基準　GPSP
Good Quality Practice　製造販売品質保証基準，製造販売後の品質管理の基準　GQP
Good Supplying Practice　医薬品の供給と品質確保に関する実践規範　GSP
Good Vigilance Practice　製造販売後安全管理の基準　GVP
governmental certificate test　国家検定
grade point average　学生の成績評価方式の1つ
graduated cylinder　メスシリンダー
Gradumet　グラデュメット製剤(放出制御製剤の1つ)
graft versus host disease　移植片対宿主病　GVHD
Gram stain　グラム染色
granules　顆粒剤
greenhouse effect　温室効果
grinding　粉砕
Gross Domestic Product　国内総生産　GDP
Gross National Product　国民総生産　GNP

H

halo effect　ハロー効果(後光効果)
hand antisepsis　手指消毒
hapten　不完全抗原
harassment　嫌がらせ
hard capsules　硬カプセル剤

hard fat 硬脂肪基剤
hardness 硬度
hazard ratio ハザード比　HR
health care 医療
health care administration 保健管理，健康管理
health care cost（health expenditure） 医療費
health care information technologists 医療情報技師
health care insurance system 医療保険制度
health care provider 医療提供施設
health care services under insurance 保険医療
health care system for the elderly 高齢者医療制度
health economics 医療経済学
health expenditure 医療費，保健費用
health impairment 健康被害
health information 医療情報
health information management 診療情報管理
health insurance 健康保険
health insurance doctor 保険医
Health Insurance Law 健康保険法
health insurance medical institution 保険医療機関
health insurance pharmacist 保険薬剤師
health insurance pharmacy 保険薬局
health insurance society 健康保険組合
Health Maintenance Organization 米国健康維持機構　HMO
Health Sciences Council 厚生科学審議会
health screening 人間ドック
healthy carrier 健康保菌者
Healthy Japan 21 健康日本21
Heinrich's theory ハインリッヒの法則
hematopoietic stem cell allograft ミニ移植，同種造血幹細胞移植
hemodiafiltration 血液透析濾過　HDF
hemodialysis 血液透析
hematopoietic stem cell transplantation 造血幹細胞移植　HSCT
heparin lock ヘパリン・ロック（留置ルート内の血液凝固防止法）
hepatic clearance 肝クリアランス　CL_H
hepatic extraction 肝抽出率　Eh
hepatocellular carcinoma 肝細胞がん　HCC
hepatotoxicity 肝毒性

herbal drugs not in the Japanese Pharmacopoeia　日本薬局方外生薬
hermetic container　密封容器
high care unit　高度治療室　HCU
high efficiency particulate air filter　ヘパフィルター（高性能エアフィルター）　HEPA filter
high performance liquid chromatography　高速液体クロマトグラフィー　HPLC
high risk group　高危険群
high risk drug　ハイリスク薬
highly advanced medical technology (treatment)　高度先進医療
Hippocratic Oath　ヒポクラテスの誓い
histogram　ヒストグラム（度数分布図）
home care management and guidance　居宅療養管理指導
home doctor　家庭医
home enteral nutrition　在宅経腸栄養　HEN
home help service　訪問介護
home medical care　在宅医療
horizontal infection　水平感染
hospice　ホスピス
hospital acquired infection　院内感染
hospital administration　病院管理学
hospital department　診療科
hospital ethics committee　院内倫理委員会
hospital information system　病院情報システム　HIS
hospital-wide voluntary reporting system for patient safety　院内報告制度
hospitalization　入院
HOT reference code　ホット番号（標準医薬品マスターコード）　HOT番号
household medicine　家庭薬
household seller　配置販売業
human immunodeficiency virus　ヒト免疫不全ウイルス　HIV
human leukocyte antigen　ヒト白血球（型）抗原　HLA
humanized antibody　ヒト化抗体
humidity　湿度
hydrophilic lipophilic balance　親水性親油性バランス

I

iatrogenic disease　医原性疾患
ideal body weight　標準体重　IBW

illegal drug(legally-obtainable incontrolled drug)　違法ドラッグ
immunoelectrophoresis　免疫電気泳動法　IEP
immunofluorescent antibody test　免疫蛍光抗体法
immunoreaction　免疫反応
immunosuppressant　免疫抑制薬
impact factor　インパクトファクター(科学雑誌の評価指標)　IF
in silico　コンピュータを用いて
in situ　生体内での
in vitro　試験管内(無細胞系や組織)での
in vivo　動物などの生体そのもの
in-country care-taker　治験国内管理人　ICC
inapparent infection　不顕性感染
incident　インシデント，ヒヤリ・ハット
incident reporting system　インシデント報告制度
inclusion criteria　選択基準
incompatibility　配合禁忌
incubation　ふ卵，培養
incubation period　潜伏期間
independent administrative institution(agency)　独立行政法人
independent data-monitoring committee　効果安全性評価委員会，独立データモニタリング委員会　IDMC
independent variable　独立変数
indication　効能効果，適応症
individual delivery　個人払い出し
induced pluripotent stem cell　人工多能性幹細胞　iPS cell
Industrial Safety and Health Law　労働安全衛生法
industry-academia-government collaboration　産学官連携
Infection Control Committee　感染制御委員会　ICC
infection control doctor　感染制御医師　ICD
infection control team　院内感染制御チーム　ICT
infection ward　感染症病棟
inflammation　炎症
influx transporter　取り込み輸送系
information disclosure　情報公開
information on proper use of drugs　医薬品適正使用情報
informed consent　インフォームド・コンセント(医師等から説明を受けた上での同意)　IC
infusion pump　輸液ポンプ

infusions 浸剤
inhalants 吸入剤
inhibition constant 阻害定数 k_i
injections 注射剤
innovation 技術革新
inpatient 入院患者
insoluble particulate matter test 不溶性微粒子試験法
Institutional Review Board 臨床研究審査委員会 IRB
insulin dependent diabetes mellitus １型糖尿病，インスリン依存性糖尿病 IDDM
insulin tolerance test インスリン耐性試験
insurance premium 保険料
insurer 保険者
Intellectual Property Right 知的所有権
intensive care unit 集中治療室 ICU
intention to treat analysis ITT 解析 ITT
interface 接点（接続部分）
interim analysis 中間解析
interindividual variation 個体間変動
intern 実習生
internal exposure 体内被曝
internal medicine 内科
internal standard 内部標準物質 IS
International Organization for Standardization 国際標準化機構 ISO
international accreditation program 医療機能評価・認定の国際協調プログラム IAP
international birth date 国際誕生日
international collaborative clinical trial 国際共同治験
International Conference of Harmonization on Technical Requirements for Registration of Pharmaceuticals for Human Use 日米 EU 医薬品規制調和国際会議 ICH
international nonproprietary name 国際一般名称 INN
International Pharmaceutical Federation 国際薬剤師・薬学連合 FIP
International Statistical Classification of Diseases and Related Health Problems 国際疾病分類（疾病および関連保健問題の国際統計分類） ICD
International Union against Cancer 国際対がん連合 UICC
internship 就業体験
interval estimation 区間推定
intervention 介入
interview form インタビューフォーム IF
intoxication 中毒

intra-rater reliability　評価者内信頼性
intraarterial injection (infusion)　動脈内注射　i.a.
intracutaneous injection　皮内注射　i.c.
intradermal injection　皮内注射　i.d.
intradermal test　皮内テスト　IDT
intraindividual variation　個体内変動
intramuscular injection　筋肉内注射　i.m.
intraperitoneal injection　腹腔内注射　i.p.
intrathecal injection　脊髄腔内注射　i.t.
intravenous injection　静脈内注射　i.v.
intrinsic clearance　固有クリアランス　CL_{int}
intrinsic sympathomimetic activity　内因性交感神経刺激作用　ISA
inulin clearance　イヌリンクリアランス　CL_{in}
invasion　浸潤
inventory management of drugs　医薬品在庫管理
investigational drug　治験薬
investigational drug administrator　治験薬管理者
investigational new drug application　臨床試験実施申請資料　INDA
investigator-initiated clinical trials　医師主導型治験
investigator's brochure　治験薬概要書　IB
isoelectric point　等電点　pI
isolation precautions　隔離予防策

J

Japan Council for Quality Health Care　日本医療機能評価機構　JCQHC
Japan Hospital Association　日本病院会
Japan Medical Association　日本医師会　JMA
Japan Pharmaceutical Association　日本薬剤師会　JPA
Japan Pharmaceutical Information Center　日本医薬情報センター　JAPIC
Japan Pharmacists Education Center　日本薬剤師研修センター　JPEC
Japan Poison Information Center　日本中毒情報センター
Japan Standard Industrial Classification　日本標準商品分類番号
Japanese Accepted Name　日本医薬品一般名称(医薬品名称調査会承認名)
Japanese Article Number Code　流通コード　JANコード
Japanese Industrial Standard　日本工業規格　JIS
Japanese Nursing Association　日本看護協会　JNA
Japanese Society of Clinical Pharmacology and Therapeutics　日本臨床薬理学会

Japanese Society of Hospital Pharmacists　日本病院薬剤師会　JSHP
Japanese Society of Pharmaceutical Health Care and Sciences　日本医療薬学会　JSPHCS
Joint Commission on Accreditation of Healthcare Organizations　医療施設合同認定機構(米国)　JCAHO
JSPHCS Certified Clinical Pharmacist　日本医療薬学会認定薬剤師
JSPHCS Certified Instructor on Clinical Pharmacist Training　日本医療薬学会指導薬剤師
JSPHCS Certified Oncology Pharmacist　日本医療薬学会がん専門薬剤師　JOP
JSPHCS Certified Senior Oncology Pharmacist　日本医療薬学会がん指導薬剤師　JSOP
judicial autopsy　司法解剖
justification reason　違法性阻却事由

K

Kampo formula　漢方処方
Kaplan-Meier's survival curve　カプラン・マイヤー生存曲線
Kawakita Jiro method　KJ法　KJ
kneading　混練
knockout mouse　遺伝子破壊マウス
Kolmogorov-Smirnov test of fit　コルモゴロフ・スミルノフの適合度試験
Kruskal-Wallis test　クラスカル・ウォリスの検定

L

laboratory data　検査データ，臨床検査値
laboratory findings　検査所見
latent infection　潜伏感染
latent tumor cell　潜在癌細胞(潜伏癌細胞)
Law against Unjustifiable Premiums and Misleading Representations　不当景品類及び不当表示防止法(景表法)
Law related to Mental Health and Welfare of the Person with Mental Disorder　精神保健福祉法
laxatives　下剤
learning strategy　学習方略　LS
legal communicable disease　法定伝染病
legal representative　代諾者

legal responsibility 法的責任
lemonades リモナーデ剤
lethal dose 致死量　LD
license for manufacturer of drugs 医薬品製造業許可
life style drug 生活改善薬
life style related disease 生活習慣病
lifelong education 生涯教育
line sepsis 留置カテーテル感染
linear regression 線形回帰
linearity 線形性
liniments リニメント剤
lipid microsphere リピドマイクロスフェア製剤，リポ製剤
liquid chromatography-mass spectrometry 液体クロマトグラフ質量分析計　LC/MS
liquid chromatography-tandem mass spectrometry 液体クロマトグラフィー・タンデム質量分析法　LC/MS/MS
liquid preparation 液剤
living will リビングウィル（死亡選択遺言）
loading dose 初回負荷投与量
local area network 構内通信網　LAN
logistic regression analysis ロジスティック回帰分析
longitudinal study 縦断研究
lot number ロット番号，製造番号
lotions ローション剤
lubricant 滑沢剤

M

magnetic resonance imaging 核磁気共鳴画像法　MRI
Maillard reaction メイラード反応
main disease 主傷病名
maintenance dose 維持投与量
major diagnostic category 主要診断群（DPCのための疾患分類）　MDC
major histocompatibility gene complex 主要組織適合遺伝子複合体　MHC
malignant 悪性の
malpractice insurance 医療過誤保険
Mann-Whitney test マン・ホイットニーの検定
market principles 市場原理
marketing specialist 医薬品卸販売担当者　MS

masking 遮蔽化
mass uniformity test 質量偏差試験
maternal transmission 母子感染
maximum tolerance dose 最大耐量 MTD
maximum drug concentration 最高血中濃度 C_{max}
maximum permissible dose 最大許容線量 MPD
maximum reaction velocity 最大反応速度 V_{max}
me-too-drug 改良型医薬品
mean residence time 平均滞留時間 MRT
measles-mumps-rubella vaccine 新三種混合ワクチン（麻疹，ムンプス，風疹） MMR
measuring glass(meet glass) メートグラス
mechanism of action 作用機序 MOA
median 中央値
median survival time 生存期間中央値 MST
medical accident 医療事故
medical certificate 診断書
medical clerk 医療事務員
medical cooperations 医療連携
medical corporations 医療法人
medical department names allowed to be indicated 標榜診療科
medical devices 医療器材
medical dictionary for regulatory activities 医薬規制用語集（ICH 国際医薬用語集） MedDRA
medical dispute 医事紛争
medical doctor 医師 MD
medical electronics 医用電子工学 ME
medical ethics 医療倫理
Medical Ethics Council 医道審議会
medical facility 医療施設
medical fee 診療報酬
medical fee schedule 医科診療報酬点数表
Medical Information System Development Center 医療情報システム開発センター MEDIS
medical inspection 医療監視
medical malpractice 医療過誤
medical malpractice information center 医療事故情報センター
medical malpractice lawsuit 医療過誤訴訟
medical office 医局

medical practice 医行為
Medical Practitioners Law 医師法
medical radiographer 診療放射線技師
medical record 診療録, カルテ
medical record management 診療録管理
medical representative 医薬情報担当者 MR
medical safety manager 医療安全管理者
medical service coverage 医療保障
Medical Service Law 医療法
medical sorcial worker 医療福祉相談員 MSW
medical specialist 専門医
Medical Subject Headings 米国国立医学図書館が定める医学科標目表 MeSH
medical technologist 臨床検査技師 MT
medical treatment plan on admission 入院診療計画
medical waste 医療廃棄物
medication compliance 服薬遵守
medication consultation 服薬指導
medication error 投薬エラー
medication history 薬歴
medication history management 薬歴管理
medicational self-understanding 薬識
MEDlars on line 米国国立医学図書館が収集する医療文献データベース MEDLINE
meniscus メニスカス
mentor 助言者
meta-analysis メタ解析
metabolic syndrome メタボリック症候群(代謝症候群)
metabolism 代謝
metabolite 代謝産物
metastasis 転移
metered dose inhaler 噴霧式定量吸入器 MDI
MHC antigen MHC抗原
Michaelis constant ミカエリス定数 k_m
Michaelis-Menten equation ミカエリス・メンテン式
micro RNA マイクロRNA miRNA
microarray 遺伝子発現差異解析
microbial substitution 菌交代現象
microorganisms 微生物
minimum bactericidal concentration 最小殺菌濃度 MBC

minimum effective concentration　最小有効濃度　MEC
minimum effective dose　最小有効量　MED
minimum inhibitory concentration　最小発育阻止濃度　MIC
minimum inhibitory dose　最小抑制量　MID
minimum lethal dose　最小致死量　MLD
minimum plasma drug concentration at steady state　最低血中濃度　C_{min}
minimum requirements for biological products　生物学的製剤基準
minimum toxic concentration　最小中毒濃度　MTC
Ministry of Education, Culture, Sports, Science and Technology　文部科学省　MEXT
Ministry of Health, Labour and Welfare　厚生労働省　MHLW
Mini Transplant　ミニ移植
misdiagnosis　誤診
missing data　欠測値
mixed billing　混合診療
mobile transport　膜動輸送
model core curriculum　モデル・コアカリキュラム
modifiable incompatibility　配合不適
molecular targeted agents　分子標的薬
moment analysis　モーメント解析
morbidity rate　罹患率
morning dipping　モーニング・ディップ（早朝の喘息発作）
morning stiffness　朝のこわばり
morning surge　モーニング・サージ（起床前後に見られる急激な血圧上昇）
mortality rate　死亡率
mucoadhesive tablet　付着錠
multi-acting-receptor-targeted-antipsychotics　多元受容体標的化抗精神病薬　MARTA
multicenter trials　多施設共同試験
multidisciplinary therapy　集学的治療
multidrug resistance related protein　多剤耐性関連タンパク質　MRP
multilayer adsorption　多分子吸着
multilayered tablet　多層錠
multiple choice question　多肢選択問題　MCQ
multiple combination　多剤併用
multiple comparison　多重比較
multiple drug resistance　多剤耐性　MDR
multiple infection　多重感染
multiple organ failure　多臓器不全　MOF

multiple regression analysis　重回帰分析
multivariate analysis　多変量解析　MVA
mutant　突然変異体(突然変異菌)
mutation　突然変異

N

nadir　最低値
narcotics　麻薬
narcotics administrator　麻薬管理者
narcotics practitioner　麻薬施用者
nasal preparations　点鼻剤
National Committee for Quality Assurance　米国品質保証委員会　NCQA
national examination for pharmacists　薬剤師国家試験
National Health Insurance　国民健康保険　NHI
National Health Insurance Law　国民健康保険法
national health service　国民保健サービス　NHS
national helathcare expenditure　国民医療費
National Hospital Organization　国立病院機構
National Institute for Health and Clinical Excellence　英国国立医療技術評価機構　NICE
National Institute of Health　米国国立衛生研究所　NIH
National Institute of Health Sciences　国立医薬品食品衛生研究所　NIHS
near-miss event　ヒヤリ・ハット事例
needlestick injury　針刺し
neonatal intensive care unit　新生児集中治療部　NICU
neoplasma　新生物
nephrotoxicity　腎毒性
neuropathy　神経障害
neurosurgical care unit　脳神経外科集中治療室　NCU
neurotransmitter　神経伝達物質
new chemical entity　新規化合物
new drug application　新薬の承認申請　NDA
new form drug　新剤形医薬品
new indication drug　新効能医薬品
no observed effect level　無影響量　NOEL
no-observed-adverse-effect level　最大無有害量(無毒性量)　NOAEL
non-clinical study　非臨床試験

non-coding RNA ノンコーディング RNA（非翻訳性 RNA），機能性 RNA　　ncRNA
non-competitive antagonism　非競合的拮抗
non-compliance　非遵守
non-conformity　不適合
Non-Governmental Organization　非政府組織　　NGO
non-inferiority trial　非劣性試験
non-insulin-dependent diabetes mellitus　2 型糖尿病，インスリン非依存性糖尿病　NIDDM
non-ionic surfactants　非イオン界面活性剤
non-linear regression analysis　非線形回帰分析
non-negligence liability　無過失責任
non-parametric test　ノンパラメトリック検定
non-prescription drug　一般用医薬品
Non-Profit Organization　特定非営利活動法人　　NPO
noncontrolled drug (legal intoxicant)　脱法ドラッグ（法律の取締りの対象になっていない薬物）
normality test　正規性検定
normalization　標準化（規格化）
Northern blot　ノーザンブロット法
noteworthy case report　重要事例情報
notification system of clinical trial plan　治験届出制度
nuclear magnetic resonance　核磁気共鳴　　NMR
nucleic acid amplification test　核酸増幅検査　　NAT
number needed to harm　有害必要数　　NNH
number needed to treat　治療必要数　　NNT
nurse practitioner　特定看護師（米）　　NP
nutrient　栄養素
nutrition support team　栄養サポートチーム　　NST

O

obesity　肥満
objective data　客観的情報　　O
objective structured clinical examination　客観的臨床能力試験　　OSCE
occupation physician　産業医
occupational health and safety　労働安全衛生
occupational therapist　作業療法士　　OT
octanol/water partition coefficient　オクタノール・水分配係数　　log PO/W

odds ratio　オッズ比　　OR
off the job training　集合教育　　Off-JT
off-label use　適応外使用
Official Development Assistance　政府開発援助　　ODA
offsetting effect　相殺効果
oil in water type　水中油型　　O/W 型
ointments　軟膏剤
ombudsman　行政監察官
on the job training　実地訓練（職場内教育）　　OJT
on-site inspection　立入検査
oncogene　癌遺伝子
one dose package　一包化　　ODP
one-tailed test　片側検定
onset　発病
open trial　非盲検化試験
ophthalmic ointments　眼軟膏剤
ophthalmic solutions　点眼剤
opioid　オピオイド，麻薬
opportunistic infection　日和見感染症　　OI
oral administration　経口投与
oral glucose tolerance test　経口糖負荷試験　　OGTT
oral transmission　経口感染
oral-disintegrating tablet　口腔内崩壊錠　　ODT
Orange Book　オレンジブック（医療用医薬品品質情報集）
ordinance of the ministry　省令
organ transplantation　臓器移植
oriental medicine　東洋医学
original medical record　原診療録
orphan drug　希少疾病用医薬品　　OD
osmolal clearance　浸透圧クリアランス　　C_{osm}
osmolality(osmotic pressure)　浸透圧　　Osm
ototoxicity　聴覚毒性
out sourcing　外部委託
out-of pocket payment　患者自己負担
outbreak　集団発生
outcome　帰結（成果）
outcome-based medical education　成果基盤型医学教育　　OBME
outlier　外れ値

outpatient　外来患者
outpatient care　外来診療
outpatient pharmacy　外来薬局
outpatient/inpatient ratio　外来/入院比
over medication(drug dependence)　薬漬け医療
over the counter drug　一般用医薬品　OTC
overall evaluation　総括的評価
overall survival time　全生存期間　OS
overdose　過量投与

P

p value　P値(有意確率)　P
P-glycoprotein　P-糖タンパク(MDR1)　Pgp
package insert　医薬品添付文書
packaging machine　分包機
paired *t*-test　対応のあるt検定
palliative care team　緩和ケアチーム
palliative care unit　緩和ケア病棟　PCU
palliative medicine　緩和医療
palliative sedation therapy　苦痛緩和のための鎮静
palliative surgery　姑息(的)手術
pandemic　パンデミック(世界流行, 汎発流行)
parametric test　パラメトリック検定
parasite　寄生体(寄生虫)
parenteral nutrition　非経口栄養　PN
partial response　部分奏効　PR
particle size distribution　粒度分布
partition coefficient　分配係数　PC
parts per million　100万分の1 (ex. 1mg/L = 1ppm)　ppm
pasive diffusion　受動拡散
past history　既往歴　PH
patent　特許
patient charge　患者負担
patient controlled analgesia　自己調節鎮痛法　PCA
patient enrollment　患者登録
patient interview　患者面接
patient medication instruction　患者向け医薬品ガイド

patient record　　診療録（カルテ）
patient referral　　紹介状，患者紹介
Patient Safety Promotion Council　　医療安全推進協議会
patient satisfaction　　患者満足度
patient treatment　　患者接遇
payment by results　　出来高払い
PDCA cycle（Deming's cycle）　　PDCAサイクル（デミングサイクル）
peer review　　ピア・レビュー（同僚審査）
per os　　経口投与　　p.o.
per protocol analysis　　PP解析　　PP
percutaneous absorption　　経皮吸収
percutaneous endoscopic gastrostomy　　経皮的内視鏡胃瘻造設術　　PEG
performance status　　全身状態　　PS
peripheral parenteral nutrition　　末梢静脈栄養　　PPN
permeation　　透過
permil　　千分率　　‰
personal drug　　Pドラッグ（EBMに基づいてよく使う医薬品）　　P-drug
personal information　　個人情報
Personal Information Protection Law　　個人情報保護法
personalized medicine　　個別化医療
Pharmaceutical Affairs and Food Sanitation Council　　医薬品食品衛生審議会
Pharmaceutical Affairs Committee　　薬事委員会
Pharmaceutical Affairs Law　　薬事法　　PAL
pharmaceutical care　　薬学的ケア　　PC
pharmaceutical common achievement test　　薬学共用試験
pharmaceutical equivalents　　製剤学的同等製剤
pharmaceutical management fee　　薬剤管理指導料
pharmaceutical manufacturer　　医薬品製造（輸入販売）業
pharmaceutical wholesaler　　医薬品卸売販売業
Pharmaceuticals and Medical Devices Agency　　医薬品医療機器総合機構　　PMDA
Pharmaceuticals and Medical Devices Evaluation Center　　医薬品医療機器審査センター　　PMDEC
pharmaceuticals and medical devices safety information　　医薬品・医療機器等安全性情報
pharmacist　　薬剤師
Pharmacist Law　　薬剤師法
Pharmacist Platform in Japan　　薬剤師綱領
pharmacodynamics　　薬力学　　PD
pharmacoeconomics　　薬剤経済学

pharmacoepidemiology　薬剤疫学
Pharmacogenetics　薬理遺伝学　PG
pharmacogenomics　ファーマコゲノミクス　PGx
pharmacokinetic/pharmacodynamic　薬物動態と薬力学　PK/PD
pharmacokinetics　薬物動態学　PK
pharmacovigilance　薬剤監視　PV
pharmacy　薬局
pharmacy practice　薬局実習
phase 1 study　第Ⅰ相試験（臨床薬理試験）
phase 2 study　第Ⅱ相試験（探索的臨床試験）
phase 3 study　第Ⅲ相試験（検証的臨床試験）
phase 4 study　第Ⅳ相試験（製造販売後臨床試験）
phenotype　表現型
photostability　光安定性
physical findings　身体所見
physical restraint　身体抑制（拘束）
physical therapist　理学療法士　PT
physician　内科医
physiological saline　生理食塩液
pillow package　ピロー包装
pills　丸剤
placebo　プラセボ（偽薬）
plan do check action cycle　PDCAサイクル　PDCA
plasma　血漿
plasma exchange　血漿交換　PE
plasma protein binding　血漿タンパク結合
plasters　貼付剤
plasticizer　可塑剤
poison（poisonous substance）　毒物
Poisonous and Deleterious Substances Control Law　毒物及び劇物取締法
poisonous drug（poison schedule A）　毒薬
pollutant release and transfer register　環境汚染物質排出移動登録　PRTR
polyacrylamide gel electrophoresis　ポリアクリルアミドゲル電気泳動　PAGE
polymerase chain reaction　ポリメラーゼ連鎖反応　PCR
polymorphism　多型性
poor metabolizer　低代謝能者　PM
population census　国勢調査
population pharmacokinetics　母集団薬物動態　PPK

portable document format　ピーディーエフ　PDF
positive defensive medicine　萎縮医療
positron emission tomography　陽電子放射断層撮影　PET
postmarketing clinical trial　市販後臨床試験
postmarketing surveillance　製造販売後調査（市販後調査）　PMS
posttraumatic stress disorder　外傷後ストレス障害　PTSD
postoperative infection prophylaxis　術後感染予防
potion　頓服
powders　散剤
powerful drug（poison schedule B）　劇薬
practical training　実務実習
preoperative autologous blood donation　自己血貯血
precaution　予防策
precautions for use　使用上の注意
preceptor　指導教員
preclinical study　前臨床試験
predictive factor　予測因子
prefilled syringes for injections　充填済みシリンジ剤
preoperative bowel preparation　術前腸管洗浄
preoperative chemotherapy　術前化学療法
prescription　処方せん
prescription bottle　投薬瓶
prescription check　処方監査
prescription drug　処方せん医薬品
prescription ordering system　処方オーダリングシステム
Prescription Privilege　処方権
prescription question　疑義照会
Prescription-Event Monitoring in Japan　日本版処方イベントモニタリング　J-PEM
present illness　現症　PI
preservatives　保存剤
press through package　ピーティーピー包装　PTP
prevalence rate　有病率
prevalence survey　流行調査（罹患率調査）
prevention　予防
preventive medicine　予防医学
price addition for breakthrough drugs　画期性加算
price of medicine　薬価
price setting by comparable drugs　類似薬効比較方式

primary care　一次医療
primary care physician　かかりつけ医
primary emergency medical care　一次救急医療
primary endpoint　主要評価項目
primary prevention　一次予防
primary source　一次資料
priority review　優先審査
privacy protection　プライバシー保護
PROBE design　前向き(Prospective)，無作為(Randomized)，オープン(Open)，エンドポイントブラインド(Blinded-Endpoint)で行う試験　PROBE法
problem based learning　問題基盤型学習　PBL
problem oriented medical record　問題指向型診療録　POMR
problem oriented system　問題指向型解決システム　POS
prodrug　前駆薬
Product Liability Law　PL法（製造物責任法）　PL法
product life cycle management　製品のライフサイクルマネジメント（製品の販売推移）　PLM
prognosis　予後
prognostic factor　予後因子
progression free survival　無増悪生存期間　PFS
progressive disease　増悪(病状の進行)　PD
Promotion Code for Prescripticn Drugs　医療用医薬品プロモーションコード
proper use　適正使用
prophylactic administration　予防投与
prophylactics　予防薬
prospective study　前向き研究
proteomics　プロテオーム解析
prothrombin time-international normalized ratio　プロトロンビン時間国際標準比　PT-INR
protocol　治験実施計画書
psychiatric hospital　精神科病院
psycho-oncology　精神腫瘍学
public funded medical services　公費医療
public health　公衆衛生
public health center　保健所
public key　公開鍵
Public Pension Scheme　公的年金制度
public-service corporation　公益法人

PubMed　メドラインデータベースの検索サービス
puncture　穿刺
pyrogen test　発熱性物質試験

Q

quality adjusted life year　生活の質を考慮した生存年　QALY
quality assurance　品質保証　QA
quality assurance unit　信頼性保証部門，品質保証部門　QAU
quality audit　品質監査
quality control　品質管理　QC
quality management　質マネジメント
quality of health care　医療の質
quality of health care management　医療経営の質
quality of life　生活の質(人生の質)　QOL
quantitative structure-activity relationship　定量的構造活性相関　QSAR
quartile range　四分位範囲
quasi drug　医薬部外品
quick response code　QRコード(二次元バーコード)　QR code
quick-release preparation　速放性製剤
quorum sensing　クオラムセンシング(安定数感知)

R

radical surgery　根治手術
radioactive medicine, radiopharmaceutical　放射性医薬品
radioimmunoassay　ラジオイムノアッセイ(放射免疫測定)　RIA
random allocation　ランダム割付け
random sampling　無作為抽出
randomization　ランダム化(無作為化)
randomized controlled trial　ランダム化比較試験　RCT
rapid eye movement sleep　レム睡眠　REM睡眠
rapid metabolizer　迅速代謝能保持者　RM
reabsorption　再吸収
readmission　再入院
reassessment system of pharmaceuticals　医薬品再評価制度
receive and inspection　検収
rectal applications　注腸剤

rectal suppositories　　肛門坐剤
recurrence　　再燃（再発）
reduction of insurance claims　　査定
reemerging infectious disease　　再興感染症　　REID
reference price system　　参照価格制度
regenerative medicine　　再生医療
regimen　　レジメン（投与計画）
regional cancer center hospital　　地域がん診療拠点病院
regional medical care support hospital　　地域医療支援病院
registered dietitian　　管理栄養士　　RD
regulatory agency　　規制当局
relapse　　再発
relapse-free survival　　無再発生存期間　　RFS
relative risk　　相対危険度
relative risk reduction　　相対リスク減少　　RRR
release behavior　　放出挙動
reliability criteria　　信頼性基準
Relief System for Adverse Drug Reactions　　医薬品副作用被害救済制度
remission　　寛解
remission consolidation therapy　　地固め療法
remission induction　　寛解導入
renal clearance　　腎クリアランス　　CL_R
repeated-dose administration study　　反復投与試験
repetab　　レペタブ（徐放性製剤の一種）
Reporting System of Adverse Reactions from health care Professionals on Drugs and Medical Devices　　医薬関係者からの副作用・不具合等報告制度
reproductive and developmental toxicity studies　　生殖発生毒性試験
resident　　研修生
response duration　　効果持続期間，奏効期間
responsibility　　責任
resting energy expenditure　　安静時エネルギー消費量　　REE
restriction enzyme　　制限酵素
retrospective study　　後ろ向き研究
reverse transcriptase-polymerase chain reaction　　逆転写酵素-ポリメラーゼ連鎖反応法　　RT-PCR
right to claim damages and losses　　損害賠償請求権
right to life and health　　生命・健康権
risk factor　　危険因子

risk management　危機管理
risk manager　リスクマネジャー
role play　役割練習　RP
root cause analysis　根本原因分析　RCA
round-the-clock therapy　24時間維持療法　RTC
Rules for Health Insurance-Covered Dispensing Pharmacies and Pharmacists　保険薬局及び保険薬剤師療養担当規則
Rules for Health Insurance-Covered Medical Facilities and Medical Practitioners　保険医療機関及び保険医療養担当規則

S

safety cabinet　安全キャビネット
safety education on medical care services　医療安全教育
safety margin　安全域　SM
salting out　塩析
salvage chemotherapy　救援化学療法
sample size　標本数　n
sanitizers　清浄化剤
satellite clinic　サテライト診療所
satellite pharmacy　サテライト薬局
scanning transmission electron microscope　走査透過型電子顕微鏡　STEM
scatter plot　散布図
school pharmacist　学校薬剤師
Science Council of Japan　日本学術会議　SCJ
second malignant neoplasm　二次癌
secondary emergency medical services　二次救急
secondary endpoint　副次的評価項目
secondary infection　二次感染
separation of dispensing and prescribing　医薬分業
severe test　苛酷試験
sexual harassment　セクシャル・ハラスメント(性的嫌がらせ)
sexually transmitted infection　性感染症　STI
shear rate　ずり速度
shear strength　ずり応力
SHEL model　シェル・モデル　SHELモデル
side effect　副作用
sieving　篩過

signal transduction　シグナル伝達
significance level　有意水準
simple diffusion　単純拡散
simple sirup　単シロップ
simple suspension method　簡易懸濁法　SSM
simulated patient　模擬患者　SP
single nucleotide polymorphism　一塩基多型　SNP(s)
single use(ad libitum)　頓用
single-blind test　単盲検試験　SBT
single-dose administration study　単回投与試験
single-dose package　一回量包装
site management organization　治験施設支援機関　SMO
small group discussion　小グループ討論　SGD
social hand washing　日常的手洗い
social insurance　社会保険
Social Insurance Medical Fee Payment Fund　社会保険診療報酬支払基金
social security　社会保障
social welfare corporation　社会福祉法人
society for investigation of medical accidents　医療事故調査会
sodium chloride equivalent method　食塩価法
soft capsules　軟カプセル剤
sorption　収着
source data(document) verification　原資料の直接閲覧による整合性確認　SDV
spacetab　スパスタブ型製剤(放出制御製剤の一種)
spansule　スパンスル型製剤(放出制御製剤の一種)
special functioning hospital　特定機能病院
special recognized medical corporation　特定医療法人
special zones for structural reform　構造改革特別地区(特区)
species difference　種差
specific behavioral objectives　行動目標　SBOs
specific gravity　比重　s.g.
specific pathogen-free animal　SPF動物(特定の病原菌を持たない動物)　SPF
specified biological product　特定生物由来製品
spirits　酒精剤
splicing　スプライシング
sponsor　治験依頼者
spray-dry method　噴霧乾燥法
stability test　安定性試験

stable disease 症状の安定 SD
standard deviation 標準偏差 SD
standard error of the mean 標準誤差 SEM
standard master for pharmaceutical products(hot reference code) 医薬品 HOT コードマスターの医療用医薬品に付与したコード HOT 番号
standard name of diseases coding 標準病名とコーディング
standard operating procedures 標準業務手順書 SOP
standard population 基準人口
standard precautions 標準予防策 SP
Standard Tables of Food Composition in Japan 日本食品標準成分表
statistical analysis plan 統計解析計画書
statistical quality control 統計的品質管理 SQC
statistical survey 統計調査
steady state 定常状態 SS
stereoisomer 立体異性体
stereoselectivity 立体選択性
sterilants 滅菌剤
sterility assurance 滅菌保証
sterility test 無菌試験
stimulant raw materials 覚せい剤原料
stimulants 覚せい剤
stock management 在庫管理
stoma 人工の排泄口
stratified allocation 層別割付
strip package ストリップ包装(ヒートシール包装の一種) SP 包装
stroke care unit 脳卒中集中治療室 SCU
structure-activity relationship 構造活性相関 SAR
Student's *t*-test スチューデントの t 検定
study and training accrediation system 研修認定(薬剤師)制度
subacute toxicity 亜急性毒性
subcutaneous injection 皮下注射 S.C.
subinvestigator 治験分担医師
subject 被験者
subjective data, objective data, assessment, plan 医療現場でＰＯＳを実践するための記載方式, 問題指向型の診療記録方式 SOAP
sublingual tablet 舌下錠
sugar-coated tablet 糖衣錠
summary basis of approval 新医薬品承認審査概要 SBA

summary basis of re-examination　新医薬品再審査概要　SBR
summary of product characteristics of ethical drugs　医療用医薬品製品情報概要
superinfection　菌交代症
superiority trial　優越性試験
supervising pharmacist　管理薬剤師
supply processing and distribution　外部業務委託　SPD
suppositories　坐剤
surface area　表面積
surface free energy　表面自由エネルギー
surface tension　表面張力
surfactants　界面活性剤
surrogate endpoint　サロゲートエンドポイント（代替評価項目）
surrogate variable　代替変数
surveillance　監視
susceptibility test　感受性試験
suspensions　懸濁剤
sustained release preparation　徐放性製剤
swallowing　嚥下
sweetner　甘味剤
Swiss cheese model　スイスチーズモデル
switch OTC drug　スイッチOTC薬
synergism (synergistic action)　相乗効果（相乗作用）
syrup　シロップ剤
systematic error　系統誤差

T

tablets　錠剤
task force　タスクフォース
teaching hospital　臨床研修指定病院
team medical care　チーム医療
technology assessment　医療技術評価
technology licensing organization　技術移転機関　TLO
telemedicine information system　遠隔医療情報システム
teratogenesis　催奇形性
teratogenicity test　催奇形性試験
terminal care　終末期医療
tertiary emergency medical services　三次救急

The Federation of Pharmaceutical Manufacturers' Associations of Japan	日本製薬団体連合会	FPMAJ
The Japan Pharmaceutical Manufacturer Association	日本製薬工業協会	JPMA
The Japanese Association of Medical Sciences	日本医学会	JAMS
the Japanese Pharmacopeia	日本薬局方	JP
the long-term care insurance	介護保険	
The Pharmaceutical Society of Japan	日本薬学会	PSJ
therapeutic drug monitoring	治療薬物モニタリング	TDM
therapeutic effect	治療効果	
therapeutic equivalents	治療学的同等製剤	
therapeutic range	治療域	
therapeutics	治療学	
thermostable	耐熱性	
Three Strike Law	スリーストライク法	
threshold limit values	暴露許容濃度	TLV
threshold limit values-ceiling value	天井値	TLV-C
tight container	気密容器	
tight junction	密着結合	
time clock	タイムクロック	
time to maximum drug concentration	最高血中濃度到達時間	T_{max}
time weighted average	時間加重平均値	TWA
tinctures	チンキ剤	
tolerability	忍容性	
tolerable imcompatibility	配合注意	
tonicity	等張化	
topical application	局所投与	
total bilirubin	総ビリルビン	T-Bil
total clearance	全身クリアランス	CL_{tot}
total parenteral nutrition	完全静脈栄養法	TPN
toxicokinetics	毒物動態学	TK
traceability	追跡可能性	
traditional Chinese medicine	漢方医学	
traditional Japanese medicine	和漢医学	
transcription	転写	
transdermal therapeutic system	経皮吸収型製剤	TTS
transduction	形質導入	
transgenic animal	トランスジェニック動物(形質転換動物)	Tg
translational research	橋渡し研究	

transporter　輸送担体
triturated powder　希釈散
troches　トローチ剤
trough concentration　トラフ濃度，定常状態最低血中濃度　C_0, C_{min}, C_{trough}
true endpoint　真の評価項目
Tukey test　チューキーの検定
tumor promoter　発がん促進物質
tumor-nodes-metastasis classification　TNM分類(国際対がん連合)　TNM分類
tutor　指導員
two-tailed test　両側検定

U

ultrafiltration　限外濾過
ultrarapid metabolizer　超迅速代謝能保持者　UM
unapproved drug　未承認薬
unblinded test　非盲検試験
unbound drug　非結合型薬物(遊離型薬物)
uncoated tablet　素錠
uninsured medical expenses　保険外診療費
unit-dose dispensing　個別セット
United Nations Educational, Scientific and Cultural Organization　ユネスコ(国連教育科学文化機関)　UNESCO
United Nations International Children's Emergency Fund　ユニセフ(国連国際児童緊急基金，国連児童基金)　UNICEF
United States Adopted Name　米国一般名　USAN
United States Pharmacopeia　米国薬局方　USP
universal decimal classification　国際十進分類法　UDC
universal health care insurance　国民皆保険
University hospital Medical Information Network　大学病院医療情報ネットワーク　UMIN
unlinkable anonymizing　連結不可能匿名化
unpaired *t*-test　対応のない t 検定
urgent safety information　緊急安全性情報　USI
usage　用法

V

vaginal suppositories 膣坐剤
vaginal tablet 膣錠
variance analysis バリアンス分析
variant 変異株
vasopressin バソプレシン
verification 検証
vertical infection 垂直感染
viscometer 粘度計
viscosity 粘度
visited medical care 訪問看護
visual analog scale 視覚的アナログスケール VAS
vital sign バイタルサイン(生体情報)
vital statistics 入口動態調査

W

ward 病棟
warning 警告
water in oil type 油中水型 W/O 型
waterless antiseptic agent 速乾性擦式消毒薬
wearing off phenomenon ウェアリングオフ現象
welfare 福祉
Welfare and Medical Service Agency 福祉医療機構 WAM
well-closed container 密閉容器
Western blot ウェスタンブロット法
WHO Programme for International Drug Monitoring WHO 国際医薬品モニタリング制度
wholesaler of drugs 卸売販売業
withdraw 製品回収
withdrawal syndrome 退薬症候, 離脱症候群 WDS
worker accident compensation insurance 労災保険
workshop ワークショップ WS
World Health Organization 世界保健機関 WHO
World Medical Association 世界医師会 WMA

Y

YJ code　　個別医薬品コード
young adult mean　　若年成人平均値　　YAM

和　名

郵便はがき

101-8791

707

料金受取人払郵便

神田局承認

894

差出有効期間
平成27年12月
31日まで
（切手不要）

（受取人）

東京都千代田区猿楽町1-5-15
　　（猿楽町SSビル）

株式会社 **じほう** 出版局

　　　　　　　　　　愛読者 係 行

（フリガナ） ご　住　所	□□□-□□□□ TEL：　　　　　　　　FAX： E-mail：　　　　　　　@	□ご自宅 □お勤め先
（フリガナ） 医療機関 又は会社名		部署名
（フリガナ） ご　芳　名		男・女 年齢（　　）
ご　職　業		

お客様のお名前・ご住所などの情報は、弊社出版物の企画の参考とさせていただくとともに、弊社の商品や各種サービスのご提供・ご案内など、弊社の事業活動に利用させていただく場合があります。

医療薬学用語集

ご愛読者はがき　　　　　　　　4576-5

1. 本書をどこでお知りになりましたか。
- □ 書店　□ 弊社DM　□ 弊社HP　□ 学会展示販売
- □ 雑誌広告【雑誌名：　　　　　　　　　　　　　　】
- □ 新聞広告【新聞名：　　　　　　　　　　　　　　】
- □ インターネット【サイト名：　　　　　　　　　　】
- □ 知人・書評の紹介　□ その他（　　　　　　　　）

2. 本書をどこでご購入になりましたか。
- □ 書店　□ 弊社販売局で注文　□ 弊社HP
- □ Amazonなどのネット書店【サイト名：　　　　　】
- □ 団体等の斡旋　□ その他（　　　　　　　　　　）

3. 職種をお聞かせください。
- □ 医師　□ 看護師　□ 薬剤師　□ CRC　□ 学生
- □ 行政関係者　□ 製薬企業関係者　□ 医療機器メーカー関係者
- □ その他（　　　　　　　　　　　　　　　　　　）

4. 本書の評価についてお聞かせください。
a. 本書の内容に対する満足度は
- □ たいへん満足　□ 満足　□ まあまあ　□ 不満　□ たいへん不満

b. 本書の価格については
- □ 割安感がある　□ 内容相応　□ 割高感がある

5. 本書へのご意見・ご感想をご自由にお書きください。

ご協力ありがとうございました。弊社書籍アンケートのご回答者全員の中から毎月抽選で30名様に図書カード（500円分）をプレゼントいたします。お客様の個人情報に関するお問い合わせは、E-Mail：privacy@jiho.co.jpでお受けしております。

0-9, A-Z

1-コンパートメント・モデル　1-compartment model
100 万分の 1　parts per million (ex. 1mg/L = 1ppm)　ppm
1 型糖尿病　insulin dependent diabetes mellitus　IDDM
24 時間維持療法　round-the-clock therapy　RTC
2 型糖尿病　non-insulin-dependent diabetes mellitus　NIDDM
2 値変数　binary variable
3-ヒドロキシ-3-メチルグルタリル補酵素 A　3-hydroxy-3-methylglutaryl coenzyme A　HMG-CoA
3,4-ジヒドロキシフェニルアラニン　3,4-dihydroxyphenylalanine　DOPA
4M-4E マトリックス分析法　4M-4E matrix analyzing method
50％最小発育阻止濃度　50% minimum inhibitory concentration　MIC_{50}
50％阻害濃度　50% inhibitory concentration　IC_{50}
50％致死量　50% lethal dose　LD_{50}
50％有効濃度　50% effective concentration　EC_{50}
50％有効量　50% effective dose　ED_{50}
5 つの R（医療事故防止標語）　five right (drug, dose, route, time, patient)　5R
5 年実測生存率　5-year observed survival
5 年生存率　5-year survival rate
5 年相対生存率　5-year relative survival
90％最小発育阻止濃度　90% minimum inhibitory concentration　MIC_{90}
ABC 分析　ABC analysis
ABC 輸送担体　ATP-binding cassette transporter (ABC transporter)
ABO 式血液型　ABO blood group
ATC 分類（解剖治療化学分類法）　anatomical therapeutic chemical classification system　ATC
BCG ワクチン　Bacille de Calmette et Guerin（仏）　BCG
C 反応性タンパク　C-reactive protein　CRP
Do 処方　ditto prescription（前回処方と同じ内容を繰り返して処方すること）
ES 細胞　embryonic stem cell　ES cell
HIV 感染症専門薬剤師（日本病院薬剤師会）　Board Certified HIV Pharmacy Specialist　BCHIVPS
ITT 解析　intention to treat analysis　ITT
KJ 法　Kawakita Jiro method　KJ
MHC 抗原　MHC antigen
P-糖タンパク（MDR1）　P-glycoprotein　Pgp
PDCA サイクル（デミングサイクル）　plan do check action cycle (Deming's cycle)　PDCA

PL法（製造物責任法）　Product Liability Law　PL法
PP解析　per protocol analysis　PP
P値（有意確率）　p value　P
Pドラッグ　personal drug（EBMに基づいてよく使う医薬品）　P-drug
QRコード（二次元バーコード）　quick response code　QR code
SPF動物　specific pathogen-free animal（特定の病原菌を持たない動物）　SPF
TNM分類（国際対がん連合）　tumor-nodes-metastasis classification　TNM分類
WHO国際医薬品モニタリング制度　WHO Programme for International Drug Monitoring

あ

アガロースゲル電気泳動　agarose-gel electrophoresis　AGE
亜急性毒性　subacute toxicity
悪性の　malignant
朝のこわばり　morning stiffness
アジア薬剤師連盟　Federation of Asian Pharmaceutical Association　FAPA
アスパラギン酸-アミノ基転移酵素　aspartate aminotransferase　AST（GOT）
アスピリン喘息　aspirin-induced asthma
アセチルコリン　acetylcholine　ACh
アセチルコリンエステラーゼ　acetylcholinesterase　AChE
アディポサイトカイン　adipocytokine
アディポネクチン　adiponectin
アドヒアランス　adherence（患者の治療への積極参加の態度）
アドレナリン受容体　adrenoceptor（adrenergic receptor）
アナフィラキシー　anaphylaxis
アナムネ　anamnese（初診時の問診・独）
アフタ性口内炎　aphthous stomatitis
アポ酵素　apoenzyme
アポタンパク質　apoprotein
アポトーシス　apoptosis
アラニンアミノ基転移酵素　alanine aminotransferase　ALT（GPT）
アルカリフォスファターゼ　alkaline phosphatase　ALP
アルコール依存症　alcohol dependence
アルコール脱水素酵素　alcohol dehydrogenase　ADH
アルサス反応　Arthus's reaction（Ⅲ型アレルギー反応の一種）
上行性感染　ascending infection
アルデヒド脱水素酵素　aldehyde dehydrogenase　ALDH
α-溶血　α-hemolysis

α-リポタンパク　　α-lipoprotein　　α-LP
アルファ 1-酸性糖タンパク　　$α_1$-acid glycoprotein　　AGP
α過誤(第一過誤)　　α error
アルブミン・グロブリン比　　albumin-globulin ratio　　A/G 比
アレルゲン　　allergen(抗原あるいは抗原を含む物質)
アンジオテンシン変換酵素　　angiotensin converting enzyme　　ACE
安静時エネルギー消費量　　resting energy expenditure　　REE
安全域　　safety margin　　SM
安全キャビネット　　safety cabinet
安全性速報　　blue letter
安息角　　angle of repose
安定性試験　　stability test
アンテドラッグ　　antedrug(局所で作用して吸収後,不活性となる薬)
アンドロゲン受容体　　androgen receptor　　AR
アンプル　　ampule　　A

い

異化　　catabolism
医科診療報酬点数表　　medical fee schedule
危機管理　　risk management
医局　　medical office
育薬　　drug rearing
医原性疾患　　iatrogenic disease
医行為　　medical practice
医師　　medical doctor　　MD
意識混濁　　clouding of consciousness
医師主導型治験　　investigator-initiated clinical trials
維持投与量　　maintenance dose
医事紛争　　medical dispute
医師法　　Medical Practitioners Law
萎縮医療　　positive defensive medicine
移植片対宿主病　　graft versus host disease　　GVHD
依存　　dependency
依存性試験　　dependence test
依存性薬物　　dependent drug
一塩基多型　　single nucleotide polymorphism　　SNP(s)
一次医療　　primary care

一次救急医療　　primary emergency medical care
一次吸収　　first-order absorption
一次救命処置　　basic life support　　BLS
一次消失　　First-order elimination
一次資料　　primary source
一次予防　　primary prevention
Ⅰ度熱傷　　epidermal burn　　EB
一日許容摂取量　　acceptable daily intake　　ADI
一日投与量　　daily dose
胃腸の　　gastrointestinal　　GI
一回量包装　　single-dose package
一般開業医　　general practitioner　　GP
一般健康診断　　general medical examination
一般名処方　　generic name prescription
一般用医薬品　　non-prescription drug, over the counter drug
一包化　　one dose package　　ODP
遺伝カウンセリング（遺伝相談）　　genetic counseling
遺伝学（ゲノム解析）　　genomics
遺伝子型　　genotype
遺伝子組み換え　　gene recombination
遺伝子診断　　genetic diagnosis
遺伝子操作　　gene manipulation
遺伝子多型　　gene polymorphism
遺伝子治療　　gene therapy
遺伝子突然変異　　gene mutation
遺伝子破壊マウス　　knockout mouse
遺伝子発現差異解析　　microarray
遺伝子ライブラリー　　gene library
医道審議会　　Medical Ethics Council
胃内容排出時間　　gastric emtying time　　GET
イヌリンクリアランス　　inulin clearance　　CL_{in}
医の倫理綱領　　ethics code in medicine
胃排出速度　　gastric emptying rate　　GER
違法性阻却事由　　justification reason
違法ドラッグ　　illegal drug（legally-obtainable incontrolled drug）
嫌がらせ　　harassment
医薬規制用語集（ICH 国際医薬用語集）　　medical dictionary for regulatory activities　MedDRA

医薬情報担当者　medical representative　MR
医薬品・医療機器等安全性情報　pharmaceuticals and medical devices safety information
医薬品安全対策情報　Drug Safety Update　DSU
医薬品医療機器審査センター　Pharmaceuticals and Medical Devices Evaluation Center　PMDEC
医薬品医療機器総合機構　Pharmaceuticals and Medical Devices Agency　PMDA
医薬品及び医薬部外品の製造管理及び品質管理の基準　Good Manufacturing Practice　GMP
医薬品卸売販売業　pharmaceutical wholesaler
医薬品卸売販売担当者　marketing specialist　MS
医薬品開発業務受託機関　contract research organization　CRO
医薬品管理　drug management
医薬品在庫管理　inventory management of drugs
医薬品再評価制度　reassessment system of pharmaceuticals
医薬品情報　drug information　DI
医薬品食品衛生審議会　Pharmaceutical Affairs and Food Sanitation Council
医薬品製造（輸入販売）業　pharmaceutical manufacturer
医薬品製造業許可　license for manufacturer of drugs
医薬品適正使用情報　information on proper use of drugs
医薬品添付文書　package insert
医薬品の安全性に関する非臨床試験の実施の基準　Good Laboratory Practice　GLP
医薬品の供給と品質確保に関する実践規範　Good Supplying Practice　GSP
医薬品の製造販売後調査の実施の基準　Good Post-marketing Study Practice　GPSP
医薬品の臨床試験の実施の基準　Good Clinical Practice　GCP
医薬品副作用被害救済制度　Relief System for Adverse Drug Reactions
医薬部外品　quasi drug
医薬分業　separation of dispensing and prescribing
医用電子工学　medical electronics　ME
医療　health care
医療安全管理者　medical safety manager
医療安全教育　safety education on medical care services
医療安全推進協議会　Patient Safety Promotion Council
医療過誤　medical malpractice
医療過誤訴訟　medical malpractice lawsuit
医療過誤保険　malpractice insurance
医療監視　medical inspection
医療器材　medical devices
医療技術評価　technology assessment

医療機能評価・認定の国際協調プログラム	international accreditation program	IAP
医療経営の質	quality of health care management	
医療経済学	health economics	
医療事故情報センター	medical malpractice information center	
医療事故	medical accident	
医療事故調査会	society for investigation of medical accidents	
医療施設	medical facility	
医療施設合同認定機構(米国)	Joint Commission on Accreditation of Healthcare Organizations	JCAHO
医療事務員	medical clerk	
医療情報	health information	
医療情報技師	health care information technologists	
医療情報システム開発センター	Medical Information System Development Center	MEDIS
医療提供施設	health care provider	
医療の質	quality of health care	
医療廃棄物	medical waste	
医療費	health care cost(health expenditure)	
医療福祉相談員	medical sorcial worker	MSW
医療法	Medical Service Law	
医療法人	medical corporations	
医療保険制度	health care insurance system	
医療保障	medical service coverage	
医療用医薬品	ethical drug	
医療用医薬品製品情報概要	summary of product characteristics of ethical drugs	
医療用医薬品プロモーションコード	Promotion Code for Prescripticn Drugs	
医療倫理	medical ethics	
医療連携	medical cooperations	
陰イオン界面活性剤	anionic surface active agents	
陰イオンギャップ	anion gap	
院外調剤	extramural dispensing	
因果関係	causal relationship	
インシデント	incident	
インシデント報告制度	incident reporting system	
インスリン依存性糖尿病	insulin dependent diabetes mellitus	IDDM
インスリン耐性試験	insulin tolerance test	
インスリン非依存性糖尿病	non-insulin-dependent diabetes mellitus	NIDDM
インタビューフォーム	interview form	IF

院内感染　　hospital acquired infection
院内感染制御チーム　　infection control team　　ICT
院内報告制度　　hospital-wide voluntary reporting system for patient safety
院内倫理委員会　　hospital ethics committee
インパクトファクター　　impact factor（科学雑誌の評価指標）　　IF
感染制御医師　　infection control doctor　　ICD
インフォームド・コンセント（医師等から説明を受けた上での説明と同意）　　informed consent　　IC

う

ウェアリングオフ現象　　wearing off phenomenon
ウェスタンブロット法　　Western blot
ウシ海綿状脳症　　bovine spongiform encephalopathy　　BSE
ウシ血清アルブミン　　bovine serum albumin　　BSA
後ろ向き研究　　retrospective study
運動療法　　exercise therapy

え

エアゾール剤　　aerosols
英国国立医療技術評価機構　　National Institute for Health and Clinical Excellence　　NICE
栄養機能食品　　food with nutrient function claims
栄養サポートチーム　　nutrition support team　　NST
栄養素　　nutrient
疫学　　epidemiology
疫学研究の倫理指針　　ethical guidelines for epidemiological research
液剤　　liquid preparation
エキス剤　　extracts
液体希釈法　　broth dilution method
液体クロマトグラフィー・タンデム質量分析法　　liquid chromatography-tandem mass spectrometry　　LC/MS/MS
液体クロマトグラフ質量分析計　　liquid chromatography-mass spectrometry　　LC/MS
エクソサイトシス　　exocytosis（細胞の開口分泌，開口放出）
エライザ法　　enzyme-linked immunosorbent assay　　ELISA
エラーの発生や波及の防止　　error proof
エリキシル剤　　elixirs
遠隔医療情報システム　　telemedicine information system

嚥下　　deglutition, swallowing
炎症　　inflammation
遠心性神経　　efferent nerve
塩析　　salting out
エンドサイトシス　　endocytosis（細胞の食作用，飲作用）
延命（延命治療）　　apothanasia

お

横断研究　　cross-sectional study
お薬手帳　　drug profile book
オクタノール・水分配係数　　octanol/water partition coefficient　　log PO/W
オッズ比　　odds ratio　　OR
オピオイド　　opioid
オレンジブック（医療用医薬品品質情報集）　　Orange Book
オレンジブック（米国）　　Approved Drug Products with Therapeutic Equivalence Evaluations
卸売販売業　　wholesaler of drugs
温室効果　　greenhouse effect

か

X（カイ）2乗検定　　chi-square test
介護保険　　the long-term care insurance
外傷後ストレス障害　　posttraumatic stress disorder　　PTSD
解糖　　glycolysis
介入　　intervention
外部委託　　out sourcing
外部業務委託　　supply processing and distribution　　SPD
界面活性剤　　surfactants
外用薬　　external medicine
外来／入院比　　outpatient/inpatient ratio
外来患者　　outpatient
外来診療　　outpatient care
外来治療　　ambulatory care
外来薬局　　outpatient pharmacy
改良型医薬品　　me-too-drug
化学受容器引金帯　　chemoreceptor trigger zone　　CTZ
化学塞栓療法　　chemoembolization

科学的根拠に基づく医療　evidence-based medicine　EBM
化学的酸素要求量　chemical oxygen demand　COD
化学的同等製剤　chemical equivalents
化学伝達物質　chemical mediator
化学平衡　chemical equilibrium
化学放射線療法　chemoradiotherapy
化学療法　chemotherapy
化学療法薬　chemotherapeutic agent
かかりつけ医　primary care physician
拡散　diffusion
核酸増幅検査　nucleic acid amplification test　NAT
核磁気共鳴　nuclear magnetic resonance　NMR
核磁気共鳴画像法　magnetic resonance imaging　MRI
確実致死量　100% lethal dose　LD_{100}
学習方略　learning strategy　LS
学術論文　academic article
覚せい剤　stimulants
覚せい剤原料　stimulant raw materials
確定診断　definite diagnosis
獲得耐性　acquired resistance
獲得免疫　acquired immunity
解離定数　dissociation constant
隔離予防策　isolation precautions
苛酷試験　severe test
過失相殺　comparative negligence
ガスクロマトグラフ質量分析　gas chromatography-mass spectrometry　GC-MS
加速試験　acceleration test
家族歴　family history
可塑剤　plasticizer
片側検定　one-tailed test
画期性加算　price addition for breakthrough drugs
画期的新薬（ピカ新）　best-in-class
学校薬剤師　school pharmacist
滑沢剤　lubricant
合併症　complication
家庭医　home doctor
家庭内暴力（ドメスティック・バイオレンス）　domestic violence　DV
家庭薬　household medicine

カテコール-O-メチル基転移酵素	catechol-O-methyltransferase	COMT
カテーテル感染	catheter infection	
カプセル剤	capsules	
カプラン・マイヤー生存曲線	Kaplan-Meier's survival curve	
顆粒剤	granules	
過量投与	overdose	
カルテ	medical record, patient record	
過労死	death from overwork	
簡易懸濁法	simple suspension method	SSM
癌遺伝子	oncogene	
がん化	carcinogenesis	
寛解	remission	
寛解導入	remission induction	
環境アセスメント（環境影響評価）	environmental impact assessment	EIA
環境汚染	environmental pollution	
環境汚染物質排出移動登録	pollutant release and transfer register	PRTR
環境順化	acclimation	
環境ホルモン	environmental hormones	
肝クリアランス	hepatic clearance	CL_H
監査	audit	
丸剤	pills	
肝細胞がん	hepatocellular carcinoma	HCC
監査担当者	auditor	
監視	surveillance	
患者自己負担	out-of pocket payment	
患者紹介	patient referral	
患者接遇	patient treatment	
患者対照研究	case-control study	
患者登録	patient enrollment	
患者負担	patient charge	
患者満足度	patient satisfaction	
患者向け医薬品ガイド	patient medication instruction	
患者面接	patient interview	
癌腫	carcinoma	
感受性試験	susceptibility test	
緩衝剤	buffer agents	
がん診療連携拠点病院	designated cancer care hospital	
がん性疼痛	carcinomatous pain, cancer pain	

完全寛解　　complete response　　CR
感染症指定医療機関　　designated infection disease control hospital
感染症病棟　　infection ward
完全静脈栄養法　　total parenteral nutrition　　TPN
感染制御委員会　　Infection Control Committee　　ICC
感染制御専門薬剤師（日本病院薬剤師会）　　Board Certified Infection Control Pharmacy Specialist　　BCICPS
感染制御認定薬剤師（日本病院薬剤師会）　　Board Certified Pharmacist in Infection Control　　BCPIC
がん専門薬剤師（日本病院薬剤師会）　　Board Certified Oncology Pharmacy Specialist　　BCOPS
含嗽剤　　gargles
がん対策基本法　　Cancer Control Law
癌胎児性抗原　　carcinoembryonic antigen　　CEA
肝抽出率　　hepatic extraction　　Eh
浣腸　　enemas
鑑定（鑑定書）　　expert evidence
寒天培地　　agar medium
冠動脈疾患集中治療室（内科系集中治療室）　　coronary care unit　　CCU
冠動脈バイパス（A-Cバイパス）　　coronary artery bypass
がん登録　　cancer registration
肝毒性　　hepatotoxicity
眼軟膏剤　　ophthalmic ointments
乾熱滅菌　　dry air sterilization
漢方医学　　traditional Chinese medicine
漢方処方　　Kampo formula
漢方薬　　Chinese herbal medicine
γ-アミノ酪酸　　γ-aminobutyric acid　　GABA
γ-グルタミルトランスペプチダーゼ　　γ-glutamyltranspeptidase　　γ-GTP
甘味剤　　sweetner
がん薬物療法認定薬剤師（日本病院薬剤師会）　　Board Certified Pharmacist in Oncology Pharmacy　　BCPOP
管理栄養士　　registered dietitian　　RD
管理薬剤師　　supervising pharmacist
含量均一性試験　　content uniformity test
緩和医療　　palliative medicine
緩和ケアチーム　　palliative care team
緩和ケア病棟　　palliative care unit　　PCU

き

既往歴　past history　PH
気管支拡張薬　bronchodilator
気管支肺胞洗浄　bronchoalveolar lavage　BAL
気管支ファイバースコープ　bronchofiberscopy　BF
危機管理　crisis management
疑義照会　prescription question
帰結（成果）　outcome
危険因子　risk factor
基剤　base
希釈剤（賦形剤）　diluents
希釈散　triturated powder
技術移転機関　technology licensing organization　TLO
技術革新　innovation
基準人口　standard population
希少疾病用医薬品　orphan drug　OD
モーニング・サージ　morning surge（起床前後に見られる急激な血圧上昇）
寄生体，寄生虫　parasite
規制当局　regulatory agency
基礎エネルギー消費量　basal energy expenditure　BEE
基礎体温　basal body temperature　BBT
基礎代謝率　basal metabolic rate　BMR
記帳義務医薬品　drugs classified as record keeping items
拮抗　antagonism
拮抗薬　antagonist
気道抵抗　airway resistance
機能性 RNA　non-coding RNA　ncRNA
機能的自立度評価法　functional independence measure
気密容器　tight container
キメラ遺伝子　chimeric gene
キメラ抗体　chimeric antibody
虐待　abuse
逆転写酵素-ポリメラーゼ連鎖反応法　RT-PCR　reverse transcriptase-polymerase chain reaction
客観的情報　objective data　O
客観的臨床能力試験　objective structured clinical examination　OSCE
キャピラリー電気泳動　capillary electrophoresis

救援化学療法　salvage chemotherapy
救急救命士　emergency medical technician
救急車　ambulance car
救急治療室　emergency room　ER
吸光度　absorbance
吸収　absorption
吸収・分布・代謝・排泄　absorption, distribution, metabolism, and excretion　ADME
吸収速度定数　absorption rate constant　k_a
求心性神経　afferent nerve
吸水軟膏　absorptive ointment　AO
急性毒性試験　acute toxicity test
吸着　adsorption
吸着剤　adsorbents
吸入剤　inhalants
救命救急センター　emergency and critical care center
居宅療養管理指導　home care management and guidance
強化療法（地固め療法）　consolidation therapy
共感的態度　empathic attitude
競合的拮抗　competitive antagonism
競合的阻害　competitive inhibition
凝集反応　agglutination
行政監察官　ombudsman
行政指導　administrative guidance
行政処分　administrative disposition
鏡像異性体　enantiomer
共同薬物治療管理業務　collaborative drug therapy management　CDTM
協働薬物治療の実践　collaborative pharmacy practice（プライマリ・ケアにおける医師と薬剤師の連携）　CPP
共変量　covariate
矯味剤　flavoring substance
共融点　eutectic point
局所投与　topical application
去痰薬　expectorants
禁忌　contraindication
緊急安全性情報（イエローペーパー）　doctor letter
緊急安全性情報　urgent safety information　USI
緊急避妊薬　emergency contraceptive　EC
菌交代現象　microbial substitution

菌交代症　　superinfection
筋電図　　electromyogram　　EMG
筋肉内注射　　intramuscular injection　　i.m.

く

空気感染　　air-borne infection
空中浮遊菌　　air-borne bacteria
空腹時血糖　　fasting blood sugar　　FBS
クオラムセンシング（安定数感知）　　quorum sensing
区間推定　　interval estimation
駆出率　　ejection fraction　　EF
苦情処理　　complaint management
薬漬け医療　　over medication（drug dependence）
苦痛緩和のための鎮静　　palliative sedation therapy
組み換え医薬品　　biotechnology product
苦味健胃薬　　bitter stomachic
クラスカル・ウォリスの検定　　Kruskal-Wallis test
クラスタ分析　　cluster analysis, clustering
グラデュメット製剤　　Gradumet（放出制御製剤の１つ）
グラム染色　　Gram stain
クリアランス　　clearance　　CL
クリニカルパス　　clinical pathway
クリーンベンチ　　clean bench
グルカゴン様ペプチド-1　　glucagon-like peptide-1　　GLP-1
グルコース輸送担体　　glucose transporter　　GLUT
グルタミン酸オキザロ酢酸トランスアミラーゼ　　glutamic oxaloacetic transaminase　　GOT（AST）
グルタミン酸ピルビン酸トランスアミナーゼ　　glutamic pyruvic transaminase　　GPT(ALT)
クレアチニン・クリアランス　　creatinine clearance　　CL_{cr}, C_{cr}
クレアチン・キナーゼ　　creatine kinase　　CK
群間比較　　comparison between groups
コース（クール）　　course

け

ケアマネジャー（介護支援専門員）　　care manager（long-term care support specialist）
経験的治療　　empiric therapy

経口感染　oral transmission
経口糖負荷試験　oral glucose tolerance test　OGTT
経口投与　oral administration, per os　p.o.
警告　warning
刑事責任　criminal liability
形質導入　transduction
計数調剤　dispense by counting
形成的評価　formative evaluation
継続的質改善　continuous quality improvement　CQI
経腸栄養法　enteral nutrition　EN
系統誤差　systematic error
経皮吸収　percutaneous absorption
経皮吸収型製剤　transdermal therapeutic system　TTS
経皮的内視鏡胃瘻造設術　percutaneous endoscopic gastrostomy　PEG
計量調剤　dispense by weight or volumetric
劇物　deleterious substance
劇薬　powerful drug（poison schedule B）
下剤　laxatives
化粧品　cosmetics
血圧　blood pressure
血液ガス分析　blood gas analysis
血液凝固因子　blood coagulation factor
血液胎盤関門　blood-placental barrier
血液透析　hemodialysis
血液透析濾過　hemodiafiltration　HDF
血液脳関門　blood-brain barrier　BBB
血液培養　blood culture
血管　blood vessel
欠陥医薬品　defective drug
血管新生　angiogenesis
血管造影　angiography
血漿　plasma
結晶化　crystallization
血漿交換　plasma exchange　PE
結晶多形　crystalline polymorphism
血漿タンパク結合　plasma protein binding
欠測値　missing data
血中尿素窒素　blood urea nitrogen　BUN

血中濃度-時間曲線下面積	area under the blood concentration vs. time curve	AUC

血糖　　blood glucose
血流速度依存型薬物　　flow-limited drug
血流律速　　blood flow limited
血流量　　blood flow rate
解毒　　detoxication
解毒薬　　antidote
解熱鎮痛薬　　antipyretic analgesics
下痢　　diarrhea
ゲル化　　gelation
原因菌　　causative organism
限外濾過　　ultrafiltration
原価管理　　cost management
減感作療法　　desensitization therapy
嫌気性感染症　　anaerobic infection
嫌気培養　　anaerobic culture
健康食品（サプリメント）　　dietary supplement
健康日本21　　Healthy Japan 21
健康被害　　health impairment
健康被害補償　　compensation for health damage
健康保菌者　　healthy carrier
健康保険　　health insurance
健康保険組合　　health insurance society
健康保険法　　Health Insurance Law
検査所見　　laboratory findings
検査データ　　laboratory data
原子吸光光度法　　atomic absorption spectrophotometry
検取　　receive and inspection
研修生　　resident
研修認定（薬剤師）制度　　study and training accrediation system
検出限界　　detection limit
検証　　verification
現症　　present illness　　PI
検証的試験　　confirmatory study
原資料の直接閲覧による整合性確認　　source data (document) verification　　SDV
原診療録　　original medical record
顕性感染　　apparent infection
懸濁剤　　suspensions

原薬　　bulk drug substance
原薬等登録原簿　　drug master file　　DMF
検量線　　calibration curve

こ

高圧蒸気滅菌器　　autoclave
抗ウイルス薬　　antiviral agents
公益法人　　public-service corporation
抗炎症薬　　anti-inflammatory drugs
効果・安全性評価委員会　　data and safety monitoring board
効果安全性評価委員会　　independent data-monitoring committee　　IDMC
公開鍵　　public key
抗核抗体　　antinuclear antibodies　　ANA
高額療養費　　expensive medical charge
高額療養費支給制度　　expensive medical charge insurance
効果持続期間　　response duration
硬カプセル剤　　hard capsules
抗がん薬　　anticancer drugs
高危険群　　high risk group
好気性感染　　aerobic infection
抗凝固薬　　anticoagulants
抗菌スペクトル　　antibacterial spectrum
抗菌薬　　antibacterial（antimicrobial）agents
抗菌薬使用密度　　antimicrobial use density　　AUD
口腔内崩壊錠　　oral-disintegrating tablet　　ODT
抗結核薬　　antituberculous agents
抗原　　antigen　　Ag
抗原結合性フラグメント　　antigen-binding fragment　　Fab
抗原決定基　　epitope
抗原提示細胞　　antigen presentation cell　　APC
交差感染　　cross infection
交差試験　　crossover trial
交差耐性　　cross resistance
交差反応　　cross reaction
抗酸化剤　　antioxidants
膠質浸透圧　　colloid osmotic pressure
硬脂肪基剤　　hard fat

公衆衛生	public health
抗真菌作用	antifungal（antimycotic）activity
抗真菌スペクトラム	antifungal spectrum
抗真菌薬	antifungal agents
厚生科学審議会	Health Sciences Council
公正競争規約	fair competition code
公正性	equity
公正取引協議会	Fair Trade Conference
抗生物質	antibiotics
抗生物質耐性	antibiotic resistance
厚生労働省	Ministry of Health, Labour and Welfare　MHLW
厚生労働白書	Annual Health, Labour and Welfare Report
構造改革特別地区（特区）	special zones for structural reform
構造活性相関	structure-activity relationship　SAR
高速液体クロマトグラフィー	high performance liquid chromatography　HPLC
酵素結合免疫測定法	enzyme-linked immunosorbent assay　ELISA
酵素免疫測定法	enzyme immunoassay　EIA
抗体	antibody　Ab
抗体依存性細胞障害	antibody-dependent cellular cytotoxicity　ADCC
高代謝能保持者	extensive metabolizer　EM
公的年金制度	Public Pension Scheme
後天性免疫不全症候群（エイズ）	acquired immunodeficiency syndrome　AIDS
硬度	hardness
行動目標	specific behavioral objectives　SBOs
行動療法	behabioral therapy
高度先進医療	highly advanced medical technology（treatment）
高度治療室	high care unit　HCU
構内通信網	local area network　LAN
効能効果	indication
後発医薬品	generic drug　GE
後発医薬品への代替調剤	generic substitution
後発品変更不可処方せん（米）	Dispense As Written
公費医療	public funded medical services
後負荷	afterload
肛門坐剤	rectal suppositories
交絡因子	confounding factor
抗利尿ホルモン（バソプレシン）	antidiuretic hormone　ADH
抗緑膿菌薬	antipseudomonal agents

高齢者医療制度　health care system for the elderly
誤嚥性肺炎　aspiration pneumonia
顧客満足度分析　customer satisfaction analysis　CS 分析
呼吸 1 秒量　forced expiratory volume in 1 sec　FEV_1
呼吸音　breath sound　BS
国際一般名称　international nonproprietary name　INN
国際栄養食品協会　Association of International Foods and Nutrition　AIFN
国際共同治験　international collaborative clinical trial
国際疾病分類（疾病および関連保健問題の国際統計分類）　International Statistical Classification of Diseases and Related Health Problems　ICD
国際十進分類法　universal decimal classification　UDC
国際対がん連合　International Union against Cancer　UICC
国際誕生日　international birth date
国際標準化機構　International Organization for Standardization　ISO
国際薬剤師・薬学連合　International Pharmaceutical Federation　FIP
国勢調査　population census
告知　disease notification
国内総生産　Gross Domestic Product　GDP
国民医療費　national helathcare expenditure
国民皆保険　universal health care insurance
国民健康保険　National Health Insurance　NHI
国民健康保険法　National Health Insurance Law
国民総生産　Gross National Product　GNP
国民保健サービス　national health service　NHS
国立医薬品食品衛生研究所　National Institute of Health Sciences　NIHS
国立病院機構　National Hospital Organization
誤診　misdiagnosis
個人情報　personal information
個人情報保護法　Personal Information Protection Law
個人払い出し　individual delivery
姑息（的）手術　palliative surgery
個体間変動　interindividual variation
個体内変動　intraindividual variation
骨塩密度　bone mineral density　BMD
国家検定　governmental certificate test
骨吸収　bone resorption
コックス比例ハザード回帰分析　cox proportional hazard regression analysis
骨形成誘導タンパク　bone morphogenetic protein　BMP

骨髄移植　bone marrow transplantation　　BMT
骨密度　bone density
個別医薬品コード　　YJ code
個別化医療　personalized medicine
個別セット　　unit-dose dispensing
コホート研究　　cohort study
コミッションエラー(やり損ない)　commission error
コミュニケーション能力　communication skill
固有クリアランス　　intrinsic clearance　CL_{int}
コリンエステラーゼ　　cholinesterase　ChE
コルモゴロフ・スミルノフの適合度試験　Kolmogorov-Smirnov test of fit
コレステリルエステル転送タンパク　cholesteryl ester transfer protein　CETP
コレステロールエステル/総コレステロール比　esterified cholesterol to total cholesterol ratio　EC/TC
コロニー形成単位　colony forming unit　CFU
コロニー刺激因子　colony stimulating factor　CSF
混合診療　mixed billing
混合ワクチン　combined vaccine
根治手術　radical surgery
根治的治療　curative treatment
根治的放射線治療　definitive radiation therapy
コントローラー(割り付け担当者)　controller
コンピュータ断層撮影　computed (computerized) tomography　CT
コンピュータを用いて　*in silico*
根本原因分析　root cause analysis　RCA
混練　kneading
コーティング剤　coating agents

さ

災害医療　disaster medicine
災害拠点病院　disaster medical center
災害派遣医療チーム　disaster medical assistance team　DMAT
催奇形性　teratogenesis
催奇形性試験　teratogenicity test
再吸収　reabsorption
細菌汚染　bacterial contamination
細菌学的検査　bacterial examination test

細菌性食中毒	bacterial food poisoning	
細菌毒素	bacterial toxin	
再興感染症	reemerging infectious disease	REID
最高血中濃度	maximum drug concentration	C_{max}
最高血中濃度到達時間	time to maximum drug concentration	T_{max}
在庫管理	stock management	
最小殺菌濃度	minimum bactericidal concentration	MBC
最小致死量	minimum lethal dose	MLD
最小中毒濃度	minimum toxic concentration	MTC
最小発育阻止濃度	minimum inhibitory concentration	MIC
最小有効濃度	minimum effective concentration	MEC
最小有効量	minimum effective dose	MED
最小抑制量	minimum inhibitory dose	MID
医薬品再審査制度	drug re-examination system	
再生医療	regenerative medicine	
最大許容線量	maximum permissible dose	MPD
最大耐量	maximum tolerance dose	MTD
最大の解析対象集団	full analysis set	FAS
最大反応速度	maximum reaction velocity	V_{max}
最大無有害量(無毒性量)	no-observed-adverse-effect level	NOAEL
在宅医療	home medical care	
在宅経腸栄養	home enteral nutrition	HEN
最低血中濃度	minimum plasma drug concentration at steady state	C_{min}
最低値	nadir	
サイトカイン	cytokine	
催吐薬	emetics	
再入院	readmission	
再燃(再発)	recurrence	
再発	relapse	
裁判外紛争解決手続	alternative dispute resolution	ADR
医薬品再評価制度	drug re-evaluation system	
細胞外液	extracellular fluid	
細胞周期	cell cycle	
細胞診	cytodiagnosis	
細胞毒	cytotoxin	
細胞毒性	cytotoxicity	
細胞培養	cell culture	
細胞分裂	cell division	

細粒剤　　fine granules
作業療法士　　occupational therapist　　OT
坐剤　　suppositories
殺菌作用　　bacterocidal action
擦式アルコール製剤　　alcohol-based hand rub
擦式手指消毒　　antiseptic hand rub
査定　　reduction of insurance claims
サテライト診療所　　satellite clinic
サテライト薬局　　satellite pharmacy
作動薬　　agonist
作用機序　　mechanism of action　　MOA
サロゲートエンドポイント（代替評価項目）　　surrogate endpoint
酸塩基平衡　　acid-base balance
産学官連携　　industry-academia-government collaboration
産業医　　occupation physician
散剤　　powders
三次救急　　tertiary emergency medical services
三種（ジフテリア・百日咳・破傷風）混合ワクチン　　diphtheria-pertussis-tetanus vaccine　　DPTワクチン
参照価格制度　　reference price system
Ⅲ度熱傷　　deep burn
散布図　　scatter plot

し

ジェネリック医薬品　　generic drug　　GE
シェル・モデル　　SHEL model　　SHELモデル
篩過　　sieving
歯科医師　　dentist
視覚的アナログスケール　　visual analog scale　　VAS
自家骨髄移植　　autologous bone marrow transplantation
地固め療法　　remission consolidation therapy
時間加重平均値　　time weighted average　　TWA
時間治療　　chronotherapy
時間薬理学　　chronopharmacology
糸球体濾過速度　　glomerular filtration rate　　GFR
シグナル伝達　　signal transduction
シクロオキシゲナーゼ　　cyclooxygenase　　COX

試験管内（無細胞系や組織）での　*in vitro*
事故　　accident
自己血貯血　　preoperative autologous blood donation
自己血輸血　　autotransfusion
自己調節鎮痛法　　patient controlled analgesia　　PCA
持参薬　　bringing medicine
止瀉薬　　antidiarrheal drugs
市場原理　　market principles
事前指示　　advance directives
持続的血液濾過透析　　continuous hemodiafiltration　　CHDF
持続点滴静注　　continuous intravenous infusion
持続投与　　continuous administration
持続皮下インスリン注入療法　　contiunous subcutaneous insulin infusion　　CSII
市中感染　　community acquired infection
市中肺炎　　community acquired pneumonia
市中薬局（地域薬局）　　community pharmacy
疾患修飾性抗リウマチ薬　　disease-modifying antirheumatic drugs　　DMARDs
実行可能性調査　　feasibility study
実習生　　intern
実地訓練（職場内教育）　　on the job training　　OJT
湿度　　humidity
質マネジメント　　quality management
実務実習　　practical training
実薬　　active drug
実薬対照試験　　active controlled study
質量偏差試験　　mass uniformity test
指定医薬品　　designated drug
指定伝染病　　designated communicable disease
指導員　　tutor
指導教員　　preceptor
自動体外式除細動器　　automated external defibrillator　　AED
自動腹膜透析　　automated peritoneal dialysis　　APD
指導薬剤師（日本臨床薬理学会）　　Board Certified Tutorial Clinical Pharmacist, Japanese Society of Clinical Pharmacology and Therapeutics
市販後臨床試験　　postmarketing clinical trial
市販直後調査　　early postmarketing phase vigilance　　EPPV
四分位範囲　　quartile range
嗜癖　　addiction

司法解剖	judicial autopsy	
死亡症例検討会	death conference	
脂肪組織	adipose tissue	
死亡率	mortality rate	
社会福祉法人	social welfare corporation	
社会保険	social insurance	
社会保険診療報酬支払基金	Social Insurance Medical Fee Payment Fund	
社会保障	social security	
弱毒化ワクチン	attenuated vaccine	
若年成人平均値	young adult mean	YAM
遮蔽化	masking	
重回帰分析	multiple regression analysis	
集学的治療	multidisciplinary therapy	
就業体験	internship	
集合	aggregation	
集合教育	off the job training	Off-JT
従属変数	dependent variable	
縦断研究	longitudinal study	
集団発生	outbreak	
収着	sorption	
集中治療室	intensive care unit	ICU
充填済みシリンジ剤	prefilled syringes for injections	
重点分析	ABC analysis	
自由度	degree of freedom	df
終末期医療	terminal care	
重要事例情報	noteworthy case report	
種差	species difference	
主治医	attending physician	
手指消毒	hand antisepsis	
樹状細胞	dendritic cell	DC
主傷病名	main disease	
酒精剤	spirits	
主訴	chief complaint	
出血傾向	bleeding tendency	
出血時間	bleeding time	
術後感染予防	postoperative infection prophylaxis	
補助化学療法	adjuvant chemotherapy	
術前化学療法	preoperative chemotherapy	

術前腸管洗浄　　preoperative bowel preparation
受動拡散　　pasive diffusion
ジュネーブ宣言　　declaration of Geneva
守秘義務　　confidentiality
主要診断群　　major diagnostic category（DPC のための疾患分類）　　MDC
主要組織適合遺伝子複合体　　major histocompatibility gene complex　　MHC
主要評価項目　　primary endpoint
生涯教育　　lifelong education
紹介状　　patient referral
消化管の　　gastrointestinal　　GI
使用期限　　expiration date
小グループ討論　　small group discussion　　SGD
錠剤　　tablets
常在菌　　flora
少子高齢化社会　　aging and low birth-rate society
消失速度定数　　elimination rate constant　　k_e
消失半減期　　elimination half-life　　$t_{1/2}$
消失率　　disappearance rate
常習者　　addict
症状の安定　　stable disease　　SD
使用上の注意　　precautions for use
消毒　　disinfection
承認申請　　application of approval
承認の取り消し　　cancellation of approval
上皮細胞増殖因子　　epidermal growth factor　　EGF
情報開示　　Freedom Of Information　　FOI
情報公開　　information disclosure
静脈血栓塞栓症（エコノミークラス症候群）　　economy-class syndrome
静脈内注射　　intravenous injection　　i.v.
蒸留水　　distilled water　　DW
省令　　ordinance of the ministry
症例検討会　　case conference
症例報告書　　case report form　　CRF
除外基準　　exclusion criteria
初回通過効果　　first pass effect
初回負荷投与量　　loading dose
除去率　　extraction ratio
除菌率　　bacterial eradication rate

食塩価法	sodium chloride equivalent method
食事療法	diet therapy
食中毒	food poisoning
助言者	mentor
照射線量	dose of radiation
初診時の問診（アナムネ）	first medical interview
処方オーダリングシステム	prescription ordering system
処方監査	prescription check
処方権	Prescription Privilege
徐放性製剤	sustained release preparation
処方せん	prescription
処方せん医薬品	prescription drug
自律神経	autonomic nerve
シロップ剤	syrup
新医薬品再審査概要	summary basis of re-examination　SBR
新医薬品承認審査概要	summary basis of approval　SBA
新規化合物	new chemical entity
新規生合成	de novo synthesis
心胸郭比	cardiothoracic ratio　CTR
腎クリアランス	renal clearance　CL_R
神経障害	neuropathy
心係数	cardiac index　CI
神経伝達物質	neurotransmitter
介護	care
心血管造影	cardioangiography　CAG
進行癌	advanced cancer
新興感染症	emerging infectious disease
人工心肺	cardiopulmonary bypass　CPB
人工唾液	artificial saliva
人工多能性幹細胞	induced pluripotent stem cell　iPS cell
人口動態調査	vital statistics
新効能医薬品	new indication drug
人工の排泄口	stoma
人口ピラミッド	age pyramid
浸剤	infusions
新剤形医薬品	new form drug
深在静脈血栓症	deep vein thrombosis　DVT
新三種混合ワクチン（麻疹，ムンプス，風疹）	measles-mumps-rubella vaccine　MMR

人種差　　　ethnic differences
浸潤　　　invasion
親水性親油性バランス　　　hydrophilic lipophilic balance
新生経路　　　de novo pathway
新生児集中治療部　　　neonatal intensive care unit　　　NICU
新生物　　　neoplasma
新鮮凍結血漿　　　fresh frozen plasma　　　FFP
迅速代謝能保持者　　　rapid metabolizer　　　RM
身体所見　　　physical findings
身体抑制（拘束）　　　physical restraint
深達性Ⅱ度熱傷　　　deep dermal burn
診断　　　diagnosis　　　Dx
診断群分類（包括医療評価制度における）　　　diagnosis procedure combination　　　DPC
診断群別包括支払方式　　　diagnosis related group/prospective payment system　　　DRG/PPS
診断支援システム　　　diagnostic support system
診断書　　　medical certificate
診断薬　　　diagnostic drug
心電図　　　electrocardiogram　　　ECG
浸透圧　　　osmolality（osmotic pressure）　　　Osm
浸透圧クリアランス　　　osmolal clearance　　　C_{osm}
（未承認薬の）人道的使用　　　compassionate use　　　CU
腎毒性　　　nephrotoxicity
真の評価項目　　　true endpoint
心肺蘇生　　　cardiopulmonary resuscitation　　　CPR
心肺停止　　　cardiopulmonary arrest　　　CPA
心拍出量　　　cardiac output
心房性ナトリウム利尿ペプチド　　　atrial natriuretic peptide　　　ANP
新薬の承認申請　　　new drug application　　　NDA
信頼区間　　　confidence interval　　　CI
信頼性基準　　　reliability criteria
信頼性保証部門（品質保証部門）　　　quality assurance unit　　　QAU
診療アウトカム評価　　　clinical outcome evaluation
診療科　　　hospital department
診療ガイドライン　　　clinical practice guideline
診療録（カルテ）　　　medical record, patient record
診療圏　　　catchment area
診療所　　　clinics
診療情報開示　　　disclosure of patient information

診療情報管理　health information management
診療評価　clinical audit
診療放射線技師　medical radiographer
診療報酬　medical fee
診療報酬点数表　fee schedule for medical services
診療録開示　disclosure of medical records
診療録管理　medical record management
心理療法（カウンセリング）　counseling
親和性　affinity

す

スイスチーズモデル　Swiss cheese model
水中油型　oil in water type　O/W型
垂直感染　vertical infection
スイッチOTC薬　switch OTC drug
推算糸球体濾過量　estimated glomerular filtration rate　eGFR
随伴症状　accessory symptom
水平感染　horizontal infection
スチューデントのt検定　Student's t-test
ストリップ包装　strip package（ヒートシール包装の一種）　SP包装
スパスタブ型製剤　spacetab（放出制御製剤の一種）
スパンスル型製剤　spansule（放出制御製剤の一種）
スプライシング　splicing
ずり応力　shear strength
ずり速度　shear rate
スリーストライク法　Three Strike Law

せ

生化学的効果修飾　biochemical modulation
成果基盤型医学教育　outcome-based medical education　OBME
生活改善薬　life style drug
生活習慣病　life style related disease
生活の質（人生の質）　quality of life　QOL
生活の質を考慮した生存年　quality adjusted life year　QALY
性感染症　sexually transmitted infection　STI
正規性検定　normality test

静菌作用　　bacteriostatic action
制限酵素　　restriction enzyme
性差　　gender differences
製剤　　formulation
製剤学的同等製剤　　pharmaceutical equivalents
制酸薬　　antacids
清浄化剤　　sanitizers
生殖発生毒性試験　　reproductive and developmental toxicity studies
精神科専門薬剤師（日本病院薬剤師会）　　Board Certified Psychiatric Pharmacy Specialist　　BCPPS
精神科病院　　psychiatric hospital
精神科薬物療法認定薬剤師（日本病院薬剤師会）　　Board Certified Pharmacist in Psychiatric Pharmacy　　BCPPP
精神腫瘍学　　psycho-oncology
精神障害の診断と統計の手引き　　diagnostic and statistical manual of mental disorders　　DSM
精神保健福祉法　　Law related to Mental Health and Welfare of the Person with Mental Disorder
製造年月日　　date of manufacture
製造番号　　lot number
製造販売後安全管理の基準　　Good Vigilance Practice　　GVP
製造販売後調査（市販後調査）　　postmarketing surveillance　　PMS
製造販売承認申請　　application for the manufacture and sales approval
製造販売品質保証基準（製造販売後の品質管理の基準）　　Good Quality Practice　　GQP
生存期間中央値　　median survival time　　MST
生体内での　　*in situ*
制吐薬　　antiemetics
製品回収　　withdraw
製品のライフサイクルマネジメント（製品の販売推移）　　product life cycle management　　PLM
政府開発援助　　Official Development Assistance　　ODA
生物化学的酸素要求量　　biochemical oxygen demand　　BOD
生物学的偽陽性　　biological false positive　　BFP
生物学的指標　　biomarker
生物学的製剤基準　　minimum requirements for biological products
生物学的同等性　　bioequivalence　　BE
生物学的半減期　　biological half-life
生物学的封じ込め　　biological containment

生物学的利用能	bioavailability
生物由来製品	biological products
成分栄養	elemental diet　ED
生命・健康権	right to life and health
生命倫理	bioethics
生理食塩液	physiological saline
政令	cabinet order
世界医師会	World Medical Association　WMA
世界保健機関	World Health Organization　WHO
脊髄腔内注射	intrathecal injection　i.t.
責任	responsibility
セクシャル・ハラスメント（性的嫌がらせ）	sexual harassment
舌下錠	sublingual tablet
赤血球沈降速度	erythrocyte sedimentation rate　ESR
接触阻害	contact inhibition
絶対リスク減少	absolute risk reduction
接点（接続部分）	interface
説明責任	accountability
セロトニン	5-hydroxytryptamine（serotonin）　5-HT
前駆薬	prodrug
線形回帰	linear regression
線形性	linearity
煎剤	decoctions
潜在癌細胞（潜伏癌細胞）	latent tumor cell
穿刺	puncture
洗浄剤	detergents
染色体	chromosome
先進医療	advanced medical care
全身クリアランス	total clearance　CL_{tot}
全身状態	performance status　PS
全生存期間	overall survival time　OS
選択基準	inclusion criteria
全日本病院協会	All Japan Hospital Association　AJHA
先発医薬品	brand-name drug
潜伏感染	latent infection
潜伏期間	incubation period
千分率	permil　‰
専門医	medical specialist

専門看護師　certified nurse specialist　CNS
前臨床試験　preclinical study

そ

増悪（病状の進行）　progressive disease　PD
相加作用　additive action
総括的評価　overall evaluation
相関係数　correlation coefficient　r
臓器移植　organ transplantation
早期臨床体験学習　early exposure
造血幹細胞移植　hematopoietic stem cell transplantation　HSCT
総合医　general physician
奏効期間　response duration
相殺効果　offsetting effect
走査透過型電子顕微鏡　scanning transmission electron microscope　STEM
相乗効果（相乗作用）　synergism（synergistic action）
相対危険度　relative risk
相対リスク減少　relative risk reduction　RRR
総ビリルビン　total bilirubin　T-Bil
総分岐鎖アミノ酸/チロシンモル比　branched-chain amino acid and tyrosine molar ratio　BTR
層別割付　stratified allocation
相補的DNA　complementary DNA　cDNA
創薬　drug development
阻害定数　inhibition constant　k_i
促進拡散　facilitated diffusion
速放性製剤　quick-release preparation
素錠　uncoated tablet
速乾性擦式消毒薬　waterless antiseptic agent
損害賠償　compensation for damages
損害賠償請求権　right to claim damages and losses
尊厳死　death with dignity

た

第I相試験（臨床薬理試験）　phase 1 study
退院時療養計画書　explaining treatment plan on discharge

退院要約（退院時サマリー）	discharge summary	
対応のある t 検定	paired *t*-test	
対応のない t 検定	unpaired *t*-test	
体外被曝	external exposure	
大学教員資質開発	faculty development	FD
体格指数	body mass index	BMI
大学病院医療情報ネットワーク	University hospital Medical Information Network	UMIN
対がん米国合同委員会	American Joint Committee on Cancer	AJCC
大気汚染	air pollution	
第Ⅲ相試験（検証的臨床試験）	phase 3 study	
体脂肪率	body fat percentage	BFP
代謝	metabolism	
代謝産物	metabolite	
対照群	control group	
対小児安全包装	child-resistant packaging	CRP
対照薬	control drug	
対診	consultation	
代替医療	alternative medicine	
代替調剤	drug substitution	
代替変数	surrogate variable	
代諾者	legal representative	
耐糖能試験	glucose tolerance test	GTT
第Ⅱ相試験（探索的臨床試験）	phase 2 study	
体内被曝	internal exposure	
耐熱性	thermostable	
体表面積	body surfase area	BSA
大麻取締法	Cannabis Control Law	
タイムクロック	time clock	
退薬症候	withdrawal syndrome	WDS
第Ⅳ相試験（製造販売後臨床試験）	phase 4 study	
多肢選択問題	multiple choice question	MCQ
多型性	polymorphism	
多元受容体標的化抗精神病薬	multi-acting-receptor-targeted-antipsychotics	MARTA
多剤耐性	multiple drug resistance	MDR
多剤耐性関連タンパク質	multidrug resistance related protein	MRP
多剤併用	multiple combination	
多施設共同試験	multicenter trials	
多重感染	multiple infection	

多重比較　　multiple comparison
タスクフォース　　task force
多臓器不全　　multiple organ failure　　MOF
多層錠　　multilayered tablet
立入検査　　on-site inspection
脱水　　dehydration
脱法ドラッグ　　noncontrolled drug（legal intoxicant）（法律の取締りの対象になっていない薬物）
ダネットの検定　　Dunnett's test
ダブルダミー　　double dummy
多分子吸着　　multilayer adsorption
多変量解析　　multivariate analysis　　MVA
単回投与試験　　single-dose administration study
探索的試験　　exploratory study
探索的データ解析　　exploratory data analysis　　EDA
胆汁排泄　　biliary excretion
単純拡散　　simple diffusion
単シロップ　　simple sirup
担体輸送　　carrier-mediated transport
耽溺　　addiction
胆道ドレナージ　　biliary drainage
単盲検試験　　single-blind test　　SBT

ち

地域医療支援病院　　regional medical care support hospital
地域がん診療拠点病院　　regional cancer center hospital
地域連携クリニカルパス　　cooperation clinical pathway
遅延型アレルギー　　delayed type allergy
遅延性過敏症　　delayed hypersensitivity
チェーン・ストークス呼吸　　Cheyne-Stokes breathing　　CSB
蓄積効果　　cumulative effect
治験　　clinical trial　　CT
治験依頼者　　sponsor
治験国内管理人　　in-country care-taker　　ICC
治験コーディネーター　　clinical research coordinator　　CRC
治験施設支援機関　　site management organization　　SMO
治験実施計画書　　protocol
治験事務局　　clinical trial administration office

治験担当医師　　clinical investigator
治験調整委員会　　coordinating committee
治験調整医師　　coordinating investigator
治験届出制度　　notification system of clinical trial plan
治験モニタリング担当者（モニター）　　clinical research associate　　CRA
治験薬　　investigational drug
治験薬概要書　　investigator's brochure　　IB
治験薬管理者　　investigational drug administrator
致死率　　fatality rate
致死量　　lethal dose　　LD
膣坐剤　　vaginal suppositories
膣錠　　vaginal tablet
知的所有権　　Intellectual Property Right
チトクロム P450　　cytochrome P450　　CYP
チュアブル錠（咀嚼錠）　　chewable tablet
中央社会保険医療協議会（中医協）　　Central Social Insurance Medical Council
中央値　　median
中間解析　　interim analysis
中国薬学会　　Chinese Pharmaceutical Association　　CPA
中止基準　　discontinuation criteria
注射剤　　injections
抽出率　　extraction ratio
中枢神経系　　central nervous system　　CNS
注腸剤　　rectal applications
中毒　　intoxication
チューキーの検定　　Tukey test
超音波診断　　echography
聴覚毒性　　ototoxicity
腸肝循環　　enterohepatic circulation
調剤　　dispensing
調剤報酬　　dispensing fee
調剤技術料　　dispensing fee
調剤報酬点数表　　fee schedule for dispensing
調剤ミス　　dispensing error
調剤録　　dispensing record
腸雑音　　bowel sound
超迅速代謝能保持者　　ultrarapid metabolizer　　UM
貼付剤　　plasters

腸溶錠　enteric coated tablet
直接閲覧　direct access
直接血液吸着療法　direct hemoperfusion　DHP
治療域　therapeutic range
治療学的同等製剤　therapeutic equivalents
治療効果　therapeutic effect
治療必要数　number needed to treat　NNT
治験分担医師　subinvestigator
治療学　therapeutics
治療薬物モニタリング　therapeutic drug monitoring　TDM
鎮咳薬　antitussives
チンキ剤　tinctures
チーム医療　team medical care

つ

追跡可能性　traceability

て

手洗い消毒　antiseptic handwash
デイ・ケア　day care
低温滅菌　cold sterilization
定常状態　steady state　SS
定常状態最低血中濃度　trough concentration　C_0, C_{min}, C_{trough}
定常状態平均薬物濃度　average drug concentration at steady state　$C_{ss\ av}$
ディスポーザブル製剤　disposables
訂正死亡率　adjusted death rate
低代謝能者　poor metabolizer　PM
定量的構造活性相関　quantitative structure-activity relationship　QSAR
デオキシリボ核酸　deoxyribonucleic acid　DNA
適応外使用　off-label use
適応症　indication
適格患者　eligible patient
適格性（包括的な臨床能力）　competence
滴下速度　drip rate
適合　conformity
（医薬品の）適正使用　appropriate use of drug

適正使用　proper use
出来高払い　payment by results
出来高払い制度　fee-for-service system
デミングサイクル（PDCAサイクル）　Deming's cycle
転移　metastasis
添加剤　additives, excipients
点眼剤　ophthalmic solutions
電気泳動　electrophoresis
電気化学検出器　electrochemical detector　ECD
点耳剤　ear drops
電子診療録　electronic medical record　EMR
電子スピン共鳴　electron spin resonance　ESR
電子データ収集　electronic data capture　EDC
転写　transcription
天井値　threshold limit values-ceiling value　TLV-C
点滴　drip infusion　DI
点鼻剤　nasal preparations

と

同意　assent
糖衣錠　sugar-coated tablet
透過　permeation
統計解析計画書　statistical analysis plan
統計調査　statistical survey
統計的品質管理　statistical quality control　SQC
同種造血幹細胞移植　hematopoietic stem cell allograft
同種同効薬　comparable drug
糖新生　gluconeogenesis
透析　dialysis
到着時死亡　dead on arrival　DOA
等張化　tonicity
疼痛表情評価スケール　face pain rating scale
等電点　isoelectric point　pI
同等性試験　equivalence trial
糖尿病　diabetes mellitus　DM
動物などの生体そのもの　*in vivo*
動脈血酸素分圧　arterial O_2 pressure　Pa_{O_2}

動脈血酸素飽和度	arterial O$_2$ saturation	Sa$_{O_2}$
動脈血二酸化炭素分圧	arterial CO$_2$ pressure	Pa$_{CO_2}$
動脈内注射	intraarterial injection（infusion）	i.a.

投薬エラー　medication error
投薬瓶　prescription bottle
東洋医学　oriental medicine
投与期間　dosing period
投与計画　dosage regimen
投与剤形　dosage form
投与設計　dosage design
特定医療法人　special recognized medical corporation
特定看護師（米）　nurse practitioner　NP
特定機能病院　advanced treatment hospital, special functioning hospital
特定疾患　designated disease
特定生物由来製品　specified biological product
特定非営利活動法人　Non-Profit Organization　NPO
特定保健用食品　food for specified health uses
毒物　poison（poisonous substance）
毒物及び劇物取締法　Poisonous and Deleterious Substances Control Law
毒物動態学　toxicokinetics　TK
匿名化　anonymizing
毒薬　poisonous drug（poison schedule A）
独立行政法人　independent administrative institution（agency）
独立データモニタリング委員会　independent data-monitoring committee　IDMC
独立変数　independent variable
特許　patent
突然変異　mutation
突然変異体（突然変異菌）　mutant
塗布量の単位　finger tip unit　FTU
ドライシロップ　dry syrup　DS
ドラッグ・ラグ（医薬品承認審査遅滞）　drug lag
トラフ濃度　trough concentration　C_0, C_{min}, C_{trough}
トランスジェニック動物（形質転換動物）　transgenic animal　Tg
鳥インフルエンザ　avian influenza
取り込み輸送系　influx transporter
トローチ剤　troches
頓服　potion
頓用　single use（ad libitum）

な

内因性交感神経刺激作用　intrinsic sympathomimetic activity　ISA
内科　internal medicine
内科医　physician
内視鏡下手術　endoscopic operation（surgery）
内的妥当性　content validity
内毒素　endotoxin
内部標準物質　internal standard　IS
軟カプセル剤　soft capsules
軟膏剤　ointments

に

二次癌　second malignant neoplasm
二次感染　secondary infection
二次救急　secondary emergency medical services
二次救命処置　advanced cardiovascular life support　ACLS
二重安全装置　failsafe
二重エネルギーX線吸収測定法　dual energy x-ray absorptiometry　DEXA法
二重盲検試験　double blind test　DBT
二重盲検比較試験　double blind controlled trial
にせ薬　counterfeit drug
二相性気道陽圧　bi-levels of positive airway pressures　BiPAP
日常生活動作　activities of daily living　ADL
日常的手洗い　social hand washing
日内変動　circadian rhythm
日米EU医薬品規制調和国際会議　International Conference of Harmonization on Technical Requirements for Registration of Pharmaceuticals for Human Use　ICH
日本医学会　The Japanese Association of Medical Sciences　JAMS
日本医師会　Japan Medical Association　JMA
日本医薬情報センター　Japan Pharmaceutical Information Center　JAPIC
日本医薬品一般名称（医薬品名称調査会承認名）　Japanese Accepted Name
日本医療機能評価機構　Japan Council for Quality Health Care　JCQHC
日本医療薬学会　Japanese Society of Pharmaceutical Health Care and Sciences　JSPHCS
日本医療薬学会がん指導薬剤師　JSPHCS Certified Senior Oncology Pharmacist　JSOP
日本医療薬学会がん専門薬剤師　JSPHCS Certified Oncology Pharmacist　JOP
日本医療薬学会指導薬剤師　JSPHCS Certified Instructor on Clinical Pharmacist Training

日本医療薬学会認定薬剤師　　JSPHCS Certified Clinical Pharmacist
日本学術会議　　Science Council of Japan　　SCJ
日本看護協会　　Japanese Nursing Association　　JNA
日本工業規格　　Japanese Industrial Standard　　JIS
日本食品標準成分表　　Standard Tables of Food Composition in Japan
日本製薬工業協会　　The Japan Pharmaceutical Manufacturers Association　　JPMA
日本製薬団体連合会　　The Federation of Pharmaceutical Manufacturers' Associations of Japan　　FPMAJ
日本中毒情報センター　　Japan Poison Information Center
日本版処方イベントモニタリング　　Prescription-Event Monitoring in Japan　　J-PEM
日本病院会　　Japan Hospital Association
日本病院薬剤師会　　Japanese Society of Hospital Pharmacists　　JSHP
日本標準商品分類番号　　Japan Standard Industrial Classification
日本薬学会　　The Pharmaceutical Society of Japan　　PSJ
日本薬剤師会　　Japan Pharmaceutical Association　　JPA
日本薬剤師研修センター　　Japan Pharmacists Education Center　　JPEC
日本薬局方　　the Japanese Pharmacopeia　　JP
日本薬局方外医薬品　　drugs not in the Japanese Pharmacopoeia
日本薬局方外生薬　　herbal drugs not in the Japanese Pharmacopoeia
日本臨床薬理学会　　Japanese Society of Clinical Pharmacology and Therapeutics
入院　　admission, hospitalization
入院患者　　inpatient
入院診療計画　　medical treatment plan on admission
入院日　　date of admission
osmolality（osmotic pressure）　　emulsifiers
乳剤　　emulsions
配合変化　　compatibility
人間ドック　　health screening
認定 CRC（日本臨床薬理学会）　　Board Certified Clinical Research Coodinator, Japanese Society of Clinical Pharmacology and Therapeutics
認定医　　certified physician or surgeon
認定薬剤師（日本臨床薬理学会）　　Board Certified Clinical Pharmacist, Japanese Society of Clinical Pharmacology and Therapeutics
妊婦・授乳婦専門薬剤師（日本病院薬剤師会）　　Board Certified Pharmacy Specialist in Pharmacotherapy during Pregnancy and Lactation　　BCPSPPL
妊婦・授乳婦薬物療法認定薬剤師（日本病院薬剤師会）　　Board Certified Pharmacist in Pharmacotherapy during Pregnancy and Lactation　　BCPPPL
忍容性　　tolerability

ね

粘度　viscosity
粘度計　viscometer
年齢調整死亡率　age-adjusted death rate

の

脳死　brain death
脳神経外科集中治療室　neurosurgical care unit　NCU
脳脊髄液　cerebrospinal fluid　CSF
脳脊髄液関門　brain cerebrospinal fluid barrier　BCSFB
脳卒中集中治療室　stroke care unit　SCU
能動免疫　active immunity
能動輸送　active transport
脳波　electroencephalogram　EEG
農薬　agricultural chemicals
ノンコーディング RNA（非翻訳性 RNA）　non-coding RNA　ncRNA
ノンパラメトリック検定　non-parametric test
ノーザンブロット法　Northern blot　NB

は

バイアス（偏り）　bias
バイオクリーンルーム　biological clean room
バイオ後続品　bio-similar
バイオテクノロジー　biotechnology
バイオハザード　biohazard
バイオフィルム　biofilm
背景　background
配合禁忌　incompatibility
配合剤　combination drugs
配合注意　tolerable imcompatibility
配合不可　absolute incompatibility
配合不適　modifiable incompatibility
排出　efflux
胚性幹細胞　embryonic stem cell　ES cell
排泄　excretion

バイタルサイン（生体情報）　vital sign
配置販売業　household seller
排便　bowel movement
培養　incubation
ハイリスク薬　high risk drug
ハインリッヒの法則　Heinrich's theory
暴露許容濃度　threshold limit values　TLV
箱ひげ図　box and whisker plot
ハザード比　hazard ratio　HR
播種性血管内凝固症候群　disseminated intravascular coagulation　DIC
橋渡し研究　translational research
外れ値　outlier
バソプレシン　vasopressin
バッカル錠（口腔剤）　buccal tablet
発がん性　carcinogenicity
発がん性試験　carcinogenic test
発がん促進物質　tumor promoter
発がん物質　carcinogen
発がん抑制物質　anticarcinogen
発症年齢　age of onset
発熱性物質試験　pyrogen test
発病　onset
パップ剤　cataplasms
発泡錠　effervescent tablet
ばらつき　dispersion
パラメトリック検定　parametric test
バリアンス分析　variance analysis
針刺し事故　needlestick accident
ハロー効果（後光効果）　halo effect
パンデミック（世界流行，汎発流行）　pandemic
反ドーピング　anti-doping
反復投与試験　repeated-dose administration study
バーコードシステム　barcode system

ひ

ピアレビュー（同僚審査）　peer review
非イオン界面活性剤　non-ionic surfactants

日帰り手術	day surgery	
比較臨床試験	controlled clinical trial	
皮下注射	subcutaneous injection	s.c.
光安定性	photostability	
非競合的拮抗	non-competitive antagonism	
非経口栄養	parenteral nutrition	PN
非結合型薬物（遊離型薬物）	unbound drug	
被験者	subject	
比重	specific gravity	s.g.
非遵守	non-compliance	
ヒストグラム（度数分布図）	histogram	
非政府組織	Non-Governmental Organization	NGO
微生物	microorganisms	
非線形回帰分析	non-linear regression analysis	
必須アミノ酸	essential amino acid	EAA
必須アミノ酸／非必須アミノ酸比	essential amino acids/non-essential amino acids ratio	E/N 比
必須医薬品	essential drug	E-drug
必須脂肪酸	essential fatty acid	EFA
必須文書	essential document	
ヒト化抗体	humanized antibody	
ヒト初回投与試験	first-in-man (human) study	FIM
ヒト白血球（型）抗原	human leukocyte antigen	HLA
ヒト免疫不全ウイルス	human immunodeficiency virus	HIV
皮内注射	intracutaneous injection	i.c., intradermal injection i.d.
皮内テスト	intradermal test	IDT
避妊	contraception	
批判的吟味	critical appraisal	
非病原性	avirulence	
ヒポクラテスの誓い	Hippocratic Oath	
飛沫感染	droplet infection	
肥満	obesity	
非盲検化試験	open trial	
非盲検試験	unblinded test	
ヒヤリ・ハット	incident	
ヒヤリ・ハット事例	near-miss event	
病院管理学	hospital administration	
病院情報システム	hospital information system	HIS

評価 assessment
評価項目 endpoint
評価者内信頼性 intra-rater reliability
病期分類 disease staging
表現型 phenotype
病識 consciousness of disease
標準化（規格化） normalization
標準業務手順書 standard operating procedures SOP
標準誤差 standard error of the mean SEM
標準体重 ideal body weight IBW
標準病名とコーディング standard name of diseases coding
標準偏差 standard deviation SD
標準予防策 standard precautions SP
病床管理 bed control
費用対効果 cost-benefit
氷点降下度法 freezing point depression method
病棟 ward
標榜診療科 medical department names allowed to be indicated
標本数 sample size n
表面自由エネルギー surface free energy
表面積 surface area
表面張力 surface tension
病歴 clinical history
日和見感染症 opportunistic infection OI
微量液体希釈法 broth microdilution method
非臨床試験 non-clinical study
非劣性試験 non-inferiority trial
ピロー包装 pillow package
品質監査 quality audit
品質管理 quality control QC
品質保証 quality assurance QA
ピーディーエフ portable document format PDF
ピーティーピー包装 press through package PTP

ふ

ファーマコゲノミクス pharmacogenomics PGx
フィッシャー比 Fischer ratio〔分岐鎖アミノ酸（BCAA）と芳香族アミノ酸（AAA）のモル比〕

フィルムコーティング錠　film-coated tablet
風土病　endemic disease
不完全抗原　hapten
腹圧　abdominal pressure
腹臥位　abdominal position
複合体形成　complexation
腹腔内注射　intraperitoneal injection　i.p.
副作用　side effect
医薬品副作用報告制度　adverse drug reaction reporting system
福祉　welfare
福祉医療機構　Welfare and Medical Service Agency　WAM
副次的評価項目　secondary endpoint
副傷病名　accompanying diseases
副腎皮質刺激ホルモン　adrenocorticotropic hormone, corticotropin　ACTH
副腎皮質刺激ホルモン放出ホルモン　corticotropin releasing hormone　CRH
腹痛　abdominal pain
服薬遵守　medication compliance
服薬指導　medication consultation
賦形剤　diluents
不顕性感染　inapparent infection
不斉，対掌性　chirality
付着錠　mucoadhesive tablet
付着性　adhesiveness
普通動物　conventional animal
普通薬　common drugs
フィッシャーの直接確率検定　Fisher's exact test
不適合　non-conformity
不当景品類及び不当表示防止法（景表法）　Law against Unjustifiable Premiums and Misleading Representations
ブドウ糖チャレンジ試験　glucose challenge test　GCT
ブドウ糖負荷試験　glucose tolerance test　GTT
部分奏効　partial response　PR
不溶性異物検査法　foreign insoluble matter test for injections
不溶性微粒子試験法　insoluble particulate matter test
プライバシー保護　privacy protection
プラセボ（偽薬）　placebo
ふ卵　incubation
フランツセル（膜透過試験システム）　Franz's cell

ブリッジング試験　bridging study
不良医薬品　adulterated drug
プレアボイド（副作用回避事例報告）　be prepared to avoid the adverse reactions of drugs
プロテオーム解析　proteomics
プロトロンビン時間国際標準比　prothrombin time-international normalized ratio　PT-INR
分枝鎖アミノ酸　branched-chain amino acids　BCAA
粉砕　grinding
分散分析　analysis of variance　ANOVA
分子標的薬　molecular targeted agents
文書化　documentation
分配係数　partition coefficient　PC
分布　distribution
分布容積　distribution volume　Vd
分包機　packaging machine
粉末製剤吸入器　dry powder inhaler　DPI
噴霧乾燥法　spray-dry method
噴霧式定量吸入器　metered dose inhaler　MDI
フーリエ変換　Fourier transform　FT
フールプルーフ（エラーの未然防止）　fool-proof

へ

平均在院日数　average number of hospitalization
平均滞留時間　mean residence time　MRT
米国一般名　United States Adopted Name　USAN
米国医療薬剤師会　American Society of Health-System Pharmacists（病院薬剤師会に相当）　ASHP
米国健康維持機構　Health Maintenance Organization　HMO
米国国立衛生研究所　National Institute of Health　NIH
米国疾病予防管理センター　Centers for Disease Control and Prevention　CDC
米国食品医薬品局　Food and Drug Administration　FDA
米国品質保証委員会　National Committee for Quality Assurance　NCQA
米国薬科学会　American Association of Pharmaceutical Scientists　AAPS
米国薬剤師会　American Pharmacists Association　APhA
米国薬局方　United States Pharmacopeia　USP
米国薬局薬剤師会　American College of Apothecaries　ACA
米国臨床腫瘍学会　American Society of Clinical Oncology　ASCO
米国臨床薬学会　American College of Clinical Pharmacy　ACCP

ベイジアン法（ベイズ推計） Bayesian method (Bayesian inference)
併発症 comorbidity
併用化学療法 combination chemotherapy
併用効果 combined effect
併用薬 concomitant drug
併用療法 combination therapy
ヘパフィルター（高性能エアフィルター） high efficiency particulate air filter HEPA filter
ヘパリン・ロック heparin lock（留置ルート内の血液凝固防止法）
ヘルシンキ宣言 declaration of Helsinki
変異株 variant
変時作用 chronotropic action
変動係数 coefficient of variation CV
便秘 constipation
β-溶血 β-hemolysis
β-ラクタマーゼ β-lactamase
β過誤（第二過誤） β error

ほ

崩壊試験法 disintegration test
包括医療 comprehensive medical care
剖検 autopsy
気密容器 airtight container
芳香族アミノ酸 aromatic amino acid AAA
抱合反応 conjugation
防護製品 barrier equipment
胞子（芽胞） bacterial spore
房室ブロック（AVブロック） atrioventricular block
放射性医薬品 radioactive medicine, radiopharmaceutical
放射線量 dose
放出挙動 release behavior
放出制御 controlled release CR
ホウ素中性子捕捉療法 boron neutron capture therapy BNCT
ホウ素薬剤送達システム boron delivery system BDS
法定伝染病 legal communicable disease
法的責任 legal responsibility
訪問介護 home help service
訪問看護 visited medical care

法令順守　compliance
補完医療　complementary medicine
保険医　health insurance doctor
保険医療　health care services under insurance
保険医療機関　health insurance medical institution
保険医療機関及び保険医療養担当規則　Rules for Health Insurance-Covered Medical Facilities and Medical Practitioners
保険外診療費　uninsured medical expenses
保健管理，健康管理　health care administration
保健機能食品　food with health claims
保険者　insurer
保健所　public health center
保険薬剤師　health insurance pharmacist
保険薬局　health insurance pharmacy
保険薬局及び保険薬剤師療養担当規則　Rules for Health Insurance-Covered Dispensing Pharmacies and Pharmacists
保険料　insurance premium
母子感染　feto-maternal infection
母子感染　maternal transmission
母集団薬物動態　population pharmacokinetics　PPK
ホスピス　hospice
保存剤　preservatives
保存療法　conservative therapy
ホット番号（標準医薬品マスターコード）　HOT reference code　HOT 番号
ポリアクリルアミドゲル電気泳動　polyacrylamide gel electrophoresis　PAGE
ポリメラーゼ連鎖反応　polymerase chain reaction　PCR
ボンフェローニの補正　Bonferroni correction
翻訳領域　coding regions

ま

マイクロ **RNA**　micro RNA　miRNA
前向き研究　prospective study
膜動輸送　mobile transport
摩損度試験　friability test
末梢静脈栄養　peripheral parenteral nutrition　PPN
麻薬　narcotics, opioid
麻薬管理者　narcotics administrator

麻薬施用者　narcotics practitioner
麻薬譲受証　certificate of narcotics receipt
麻薬譲渡証　certificate of narcotics transfer
マン・ホイットニーの検定　Mann-Whitney test
慢性毒性試験　chronic toxicity test
慢性閉塞性肺疾患　chronic obstructive pulmonary disease　COPD

み

ミカエリス・メンテン式　Michaelis-Menten equation
ミカエリス定数　Michaelis constant　k_m
未承認薬　unapproved drug
密着結合　tight junction
密封容器　hermetic container
密閉容器　well-closed container
ミニ移植　mini transplant
民間薬（民間療法）　mini transplant
民事責任　civil liability

む

無影響量　no observed effect level　NOEL
無過失責任　non-negligence liability
無菌　asepsis
無菌試験　sterility test
無再発生存期間　relapse-free survival　RFS
ランダム化比較試験　randomized controlled trial　RCT
無作為抽出　random sampling
無晶形（非晶質）　amorphous
無増悪生存期間　progression free survival　PFS
無病生存期間　disease free survival　DFS

め

銘柄別収載方式　drug pricing system based on brand
メイラード反応　Maillard reaction
メスシリンダー　graduated cylinder
メタ解析　meta-analysis

メタボリック症候群（代謝症候群）　metabolic syndrome
滅菌剤　sterilants
滅菌保証　sterility assurance
メニスカス　meniscus
メノウ乳鉢　agate mortar
メノウ乳棒　agate pestle
めまい　dizziness
免疫蛍光抗体法　immunofluorescent antibody test
免疫電気泳動法　immunoelectrophoresis　IEP
免疫反応　immunoreaction
免疫抑制薬　immunosuppressant
メートグラス　measuring glass（meet glass）

も

盲検化　blinding
盲検下レビュー　blind review
模擬患者　simulated patient　SP
持ち越し効果　carried over effect
モデル・コアカリキュラム　model core curriculum
問題基盤型学習　problem based learning　PBL
問題指向型解決システム　problem oriented system　POS
問題指向型診療録　problem oriented medical record　POMR
文部科学省　Ministry of Education, Culture, Sports, Science and Technology　MEXT
モーニング・ディップ　morning dipping（早朝の喘息発作）
モーメント解析　moment analysis

や

薬学教育に関する規範　Good Pharmacy Education Practice　GPEP
薬学共用試験　pharmaceutical common achievement test
薬学的ケア　pharmaceutical care　PC
薬剤イベントモニタリング　drug event monitoring　DEM
薬剤疫学　pharmacoepidemiology
薬剤監視　pharmacovigilance　PV
薬剤感受性試験　drug susceptibility test
薬剤管理指導料　pharmaceutical management fee
薬剤経済学　pharmacoeconomics

薬剤師　pharmacist
薬剤師綱領　Pharmacist Platform in Japan
薬剤師国家試験　national examination for pharmacists
薬剤師法　Pharmacist Law
薬剤師倫理規定　Code of Ethics for Pharmacist
薬剤耐性　drug resistance
薬剤溶出ステント　drug-eluting stent
薬事委員会　Pharmaceutical Affairs Committee
薬識　medicational self-understanding
薬事法　Pharmaceutical Affairs Law　PAL
薬疹　drug rush
薬袋　envelope for drugs
薬物アレルギー　drug allergy
薬物依存　drug dependence
薬物間相互作用　drug-drug interaction
薬物送達システム　drug delivery system　DDS
薬物動態と薬力学　pharmacokinetic/pharmacodynamic　PK/PD
薬物動態学　pharmacokinetics　PK
薬物輸送担体　drug transporter
薬物乱用　drug abuse
薬包紙　drug packing paper〔medicine wrapping paper, charta（ラテン）〕
薬用量　dosage
薬理遺伝学　Pharmacogenetics　PG
薬理学的協力作用を表す指標　fractional inhibitory concentration index　FIC index
薬力学　pharmacodynamics　PD
薬歴　medication history
薬歴管理　medication history management
役割練習　role play　RP
薬価　price of medicine
薬価基準　Drug Price List
薬局　pharmacy
薬局業務規範　Good Pharmacy Practice　GPP
薬局実習　pharmacy practice

ゆ

有意水準　significance level
優越性試験　superiority trial

有害事象　　adverse event　　AE
有害事象共通用語規準　　Common Terminology Criteria for Adverse Event　　CTCAE
医薬品有害反応　　adverse drug reaction　　ADR
有害必要数　　number needed to harm　　NNH
有効成分　　active ingredient
有効濃度　　effective concentration　　EC
有効半減期　　efficiency half life
有酸素運動　　aerobic training
有床診療所　　clinic with beds for inpatients
優先審査　　priority review
有病率　　prevalence rate
遊離型薬物（非結合型薬物）　　free drug
優良工業製造規範　　Good Industrial Large Scale Practice　　GILSP
輸液ポンプ　　infusion pump
輸送担体　　transporter
油中水型　　water in oil type　　W/O型
ユニセフ（国連国際児童緊急基金，国連児童基金）　　United Nations International Children's Emergency Fund　　UNICEF
輸入感染症　　afferent infectious disease
ユネスコ（国連教育科学文化機関）　　United Nations Educational, Scientific and Cultural Organization　　UNESCO

よ

溶解　　dissolution
溶菌　　bactereriolysis
溶出試験　　dissolution test
陽電子放射断層撮影　　positron emission tomography　　PET
溶媒和　　cosolvate
用法　　usage
用法用量　　dosage and administration
用量規制因子　　dose limiting factor　　DLF
用量制限毒性　　dose limiting toxicity　　DLT
用量設定試験　　dose-finding study
用量相関　　dose response relationship
用量反応試験　　dose response study
予後　　prognosis
予後因子　　prognostic factor

予測因子　predictive factor
予防　prevention
予防医学　preventive medicine
予防策　precaution
予防的化学療法　chemoprophylaxis
予防投与　prophylactic administration
予防薬　prophylactics

ら

ラジオイムノアッセイ（放射免疫測定）　radioimmunoassay　RIA
ランダム化（無作為化）　randomization
ランダム割付け　random allocation
乱用　abuse

り

利益相反　conflict of interest　COI
理学療法士　physical therapist　PT
罹患率　morbidity rate
離散変数　discrete variable
リスクマネジャー　risk manager
離脱症候群　withdrawal syndrome　WDS
立証責任　burden of proof
立体異性体　stereoisomer
立体選択性　stereoselectivity
リニメント剤　liniments
離乳　ablactation
リピドマイクロスフェア製剤　lipid microsphere
リビングウィル（死亡選択遺言）　living will
リポ製剤　lipid microsphere
リモナーデ剤　lemonades
流エキス剤　fluid extracts
流行調査（罹患率調査）　prevalence survey
留置カテーテル感染　line sepsis
流通コード　Japanese Article Number Code　JANコード
粒度分布　particle size distribution
両側検定　two-tailed test

両性界面活性剤	amphoteric surface active agents
良性の	benign
履歴書	curriculum vitae　CV
臨界相対湿度	critical relative humidity　CRH
臨床疫学	clinical epidemiology
臨床記録	clinical record
臨床研究	clinical research
臨床研究審査委員会	Institutional Review Board　IRB
臨床検査	clinical test
臨床検査技師	medical technologist　MT
臨床検査値	laboratory data
臨床研修	clinical practice
臨床研修指定病院	teaching hospital
臨床試験	clinical study
臨床試験実施申請資料	investigational new drug application　INDA
臨床指標	clinical indicator
臨床所見	clinical finding
臨床進行度	clinical stage
臨床心理士	clinical psychologist
臨床診療	clinical practice
臨床成績	clinical results
臨床的同等性	clinical equivalence
臨床病理検討会	clinic-pathological conference　CPC
臨床薬学	clinical pharmacy
臨床薬学的業務	clinical pharmacy practice
臨床薬剤学	clinical pharmaceutics
臨床薬物動態学	clinical pharmacokinetics
臨床薬理学	clinical pharmacology
臨床用量	clinical dose
倫理委員会	ethics committee
倫理綱領	code of ethics

る

類似薬効比較方式	price setting by comparable drugs

れ

冷罨法　cold application
レジメン（投与計画）　regimen
レペタブ　repetab（徐放性製剤の一種）
レム睡眠　rapid eye movement sleep　REM 睡眠
連結不可能匿名化　unlinkable anonymizing
連続携行式腹膜透析　continuous ambulatory peritoneal dialysis　CAPD
連続変数　continuous variable

ろ

労災保険　worker accident compensation insurance
老人病院　geriatric hospital
老人保健施設　geriatric health care facility
労働安全衛生　occupational health and safety
労働安全衛生法　Industrial Safety and Health Law
ろ過滅菌　filtration sterilization
ろ過率　filtration fraction　FF
ロジスティック回帰分析　logistic regression analysis
ロット番号　lot number
ローション剤　lotions

わ

和漢医学　traditional Japanese medicine
割付　allocation
ワークショップ　workshop　WS

略　　語

記号，0-9，α-Ω

‰　permil　千分率
5-HT　5-hydroxytryptamine (serotonin)　セロトニン
5R　five right (drug, dose, route, time, patient)　5つのR(医療事故防止標語)
α-LP　α-lipoprotein　α-リポタンパク
γ-GTP　γ-glutamyltranspeptidase　γ-グルタミルトランスペプチダーゼ

A

A　ampule　アンプル
A/G比　albumin-globulin ratio　アルブミン・グロブリン比
AAA　aromatic amino acid　芳香族アミノ酸
AAPS　American Association of Pharmaceutical Scientists　米国薬科学会
Ab　antibody　抗体
ACA　American College of Apothecaries　米国薬局薬剤師会
ACCP　American College of Clinical Pharmacy　米国臨床薬学会
ACE　angiotensin converting enzyme　アンジオテンシン変換酵素
ACh　acetylcholine　アセチルコリン
AChE　acetylcholinesterase　アセチルコリンエステラーゼ
ACLS　advanced cardiovascular life support　二次救命処置
ACTH　adrenocorticotropic hormone, corticotropin　副腎皮質刺激ホルモン
ADCC　antibody-dependent cellular cytotoxicity　抗体依存性細胞障害
ADH　alcohol dehydrogenase　アルコール脱水素酵素
ADH　antidiuretic hormone　抗利尿ホルモン(バソプレシン)
ADI　acceptable daily intake　一日許容摂取量
ADL　activities of daily living　日常生活動作
ADME　absorption, distribution, metabolism, and excretion　吸収・分布・代謝・排泄
ADR　adverse drug reaction　医薬品有害反応
ADR　alternative dispute resolution　裁判外紛争解決手続
AE　adverse event　有害事象
AED　automated external defibrillator　自動体外式除細動器
Ag　antigen　抗原
AGE　agarose-gel electrophoresis　アガロースゲル電気泳動
AGP　α_1-acid glycoprotein　アルファ1-酸性糖タンパク
AIDS　acquired immunodeficiency syndrome　後天性免疫不全症候群(エイズ)
AIFN　Association of International Foods and Nutrition　国際栄養食品協会
AJCC　American Joint Committee on Cancer　対がん米国合同委員会

AJHA	All Japan Hospital Association	全日本病院協会
ALDH	aldehyde dehydrogenase	アルデヒド脱水素酵素
ALP	alkaline phosphatase	アルカリフォスファターゼ
ALT(GPT)	alanine aminotransferase	アラニンアミノ基転移酵素
ANA	antinuclear antibodies	抗核抗体
ANOVA	analysis of variance	分散分析
ANP	atrial natriuretic peptide	心房性ナトリウム利尿ペプチド
AO	absorptive ointment	吸水軟膏
APC	antigen presentation cell	抗原提示細胞
APD	automated peritoneal dialysis	自動腹膜透析
APhA	American Pharmacists Association	米国薬剤師会
AR	androgen receptor	アンドロゲン受容体
ASCO	American Society of Clinical Oncology	米国臨床腫瘍学会
ASHP	American Society of Health-System Pharmacists	米国医療薬剤師会(病院薬剤師会に相当)
AST(GOT)	aspartate aminotransferase	アスパラギン酸-アミノ基転移酵素
ATC	anatomical therapeutic chemical classification system	ATC分類(解剖治療化学分類法)
AUC	area under the blood concentration time curve	血中濃度-時間曲線下面積
AUD	antimicrobial use density	抗菌薬使用密度

B

BAL	bronchoalveolar lavage	気管支肺胞洗浄
BBB	blood-brain barrier	血液脳関門
BBT	basal body temperature	基礎体温
BCAA	branched-chain amino acids	分枝鎖アミノ酸
BCG	Bacille de Calmette et Guerin(仏)	BCGワクチン
BCHIVPS	Board Certified HIV Pharmacy Specialist	HIV感染症専門薬剤師(日本病院薬剤師会)
BCICPS	Board Certified Infection Control Pharmacy Specialist	感染制御専門薬剤師(日本病院薬剤師会)
BCOPS	Board Certified Oncology Pharmacy Specialist	がん専門薬剤師(日本病院薬剤師会)
BCPIC	Board Certified Pharmacist in Infection Control	感染制御認定薬剤師(日本病院薬剤師会)
BCPOP	Board Certified Pharmacist in Oncology Pharmacy	がん薬物療法認定薬剤師(日本病院薬剤師会)

BCPPP Board Certified Pharmacist in Psychiatric Pharmacy　精神科薬物療法認定薬剤師（日本病院薬剤師会）
BCPPPL Board Certified Pharmacist in Pharmacotherapy during Pregnancy and Lactation　妊婦・授乳婦薬物療法認定薬剤師（日本病院薬剤師会）
BCPPS Board Certified Psychiatric Pharmacy Specialist　精神科専門薬剤師（日本病院薬剤師会）
BCPSPPL Board Certified Pharmacy Specialist in Pharmacotherapy during Pregnancy and Lactation　妊婦・授乳婦専門薬剤師（日本病院薬剤師会）
BCSFB brain cerebrospinal fluid barrier　脳脊髄液関門
BDS boron delivery system　ホウ素薬剤送達システム
BE bioequivalence　生物学的同等性
BEE basal energy expenditure　基礎エネルギー消費量
BF bronchofiberscopy　気管支ファイバースコープ
BFP biological false positive　生物学的偽陽性
BFP body fat percentage　体脂肪率
BiPAP bi-levels of positive airway pressures　二相性気道腸圧
BLS basic life support　一次救命処置
BMD bone mineral density　骨塩密度
BMI body mass index　体格指数
BMP bone morphogenetic protein　骨形成誘導タンパク
BMR basal metabolic rate　基礎代謝率
BMT bone marrow transplantation　骨髄移植
BNCT boron neutron capture therapy　ホウ素中性子捕捉療法
BOD biochemical oxygen demand　生物化学的酸素要求量
BS breath sound　呼吸音
BSA body surfase area　体表面積
BSA bovine serum albumin　ウシ血清アルブミン
BSE bovine spongiform encephalopathy　ウシ海綿状脳症
BTR branched-chain amino acid and tyrosine molar ratio　総分岐鎖アミノ酸/チロシンモル比
BUN blood urea nitrogen　血中尿素窒素

C

C_0　C_{min}　C_{trough}　trough concentration　定常状態最低血中濃度，トラフ濃度
CAG cardioangiography　心血管造影
CAPD continuous ambulatory peritoneal dialysis　連続携行式腹膜透析
CCU coronary care unit　冠動脈疾患集中治療室（内科系集中治療室）

CDC	Centers for Disease Control and Prevention	米国疾病予防管理センター
cDNA	complementary DNA	相補的DNA
CDTM	collaborative drug therapy management	共同薬物治療管理業務
CEA	carcinoembryonic antigen	癌胎児性抗原
CETP	cholesteryl ester transfer protein	コレステリルエステル転送タンパク
CFU	colony forming unit	コロニー形成単位
CHDF	continuous hemodiafiltration	持続的血液濾過透析
ChE	cholinesterase	コリンエステラーゼ
CI	cardiac index	心係数
CI	confidence interval	信頼区間
CK	creatine kinase	クレアチン・キナーゼ
CL	clearance	クリアランス
CL_{cr}, C_{cr}	creatinine clearance	クレアチニン・クリアランス
CL_H	hepatic clearance	肝クリアランス
CL_{in}	inulin clearance	イヌリンクリアランス
CL_{int}	intrinsic clearance	固有クリアランス
CL_R	renal clearance	腎クリアランス
CL_{tot}	total clearance	全身クリアランス
C_{max}	maximum drug concentration	最高血中濃度
C_{min}	minimum plasma drug concentration at steady state	最低血中濃度
CNS	central nervous system	中枢神経系
CNS	certified nurse specialist	専門看護師
COD	chemical oxygen demand	化学的酸素要求量
COI	conflict of interest	利益相反
COMT	catechol-O-methyltransferase	カテコール-O-メチル基転移酵素
COPD	chronic obstructive pulmonary disease	慢性閉塞性肺疾患
C_{osm}	osmolal clearance	浸透圧クリアランス
COX	cyclooxygenase	シクロオキシゲナーゼ
CPA	cardiopulmonary arrest	心肺停止
CPA	Chinese Pharmaceutical Association	中国薬学会
CPB	cardiopulmonary bypass	人工心肺
CPC	clinic-pathological conference	臨床病理検討会
CPP	collaborative pharmacy practice	協働薬物治療の実践（プライマリ・ケアにおける医師と薬剤師の連携）
CPR	cardiopulmonary resuscitation	心肺蘇生
CQI	continuous quality improvement	継続的質改善
CR	complete response	完全寛解
CR	controlled release	放出制御

CRA	clinical research associate	治験モニタリング担当者（モニター）
CRC	clinical research coordinator	治験コーディネーター
CRF	case report form	症例報告書
CRH	corticotropin releasing hormone	副腎皮質刺激ホルモン放出ホルモン
CRH	critical relative humidity	臨界相対湿度
CRO	contract research organization	医薬品開発業務受託機関
CRP	C-reactive protein	C 反応性タンパク
CRP	child-resistant packaging	対小児安全包装
CSB	Cheyne-Stokes breathing	チェーン・ストークス呼吸
CSF	cerebrospinal fluid	脳脊髄液
CSF	colony stimulating factor	コロニー刺激因子
CSII	contiuous subcutaneous insulin infusion	持続皮下インスリン注入療法
C_{ss}	drug concentration at steady state	定常状態
$C_{ss\,av}$	average drug concentration at steady state	定常状態平均薬物濃度
CS 分析	customer satisfaction analysis	顧客満足度分析
CT	clinical trial	治験
CT	computed (computerized) tomography	コンピュータ断層撮影
CTCAE	Common Terminology Criteria for Adverse Event	有害事象共通用語規準
CTR	cardiothoracic ratio	心胸郭比
CTZ	chemoreceptor trigger zone	化学受容器引金帯
CU	compassionate use	（未承認薬の）人道的使用
CV	coefficient of variation	変動係数
CV	curriculum vitae	履歴書
CYP	cytochrome P450	チトクロム P450

D

DAW	Dispense As Written	後発品変更不可処方せん（米）
DBT	double blind test	二重盲検試験
DC	dendritic cell	樹状細胞
DDS	drug delivery system	薬物送達システム
DEM	drug event monitoring	薬剤イベントモニタリング
DEXA 法	dual energy x-ray absorptiometry	二重エネルギー X 線吸収測定法
df	degree of freedom	自由度
DFS	disease free survival	無病生存期間
DHP	direct hemoperfusion	直接血液吸着療法
DI	drip infusion	点滴
DI	drug information	医薬品情報

DIC	disseminated intravascular coagulation	播種性血管内凝固症候群
DLF	dose limiting factor	用量規制因子
DLT	dose limiting toxicity	用量制限毒性
DM	diabetes mellitus	糖尿病
DMARDs	disease-modifying antirheumatic drugs	疾患修飾性抗リウマチ薬
DMAT	disaster medical assistance team	災害派遣医療チーム
DMF	drug master file	原薬等登録原簿
DNA	deoxyribonucleic acid	デオキシリボ核酸
DOA	dead on arrival	到着時死亡
DOPA	3,4-dihydroxyphenylalanine	3,4-ジヒドロキシフェニルアラニン
DPC	diagnosis procedure combination	診断群分類（包括医療評価制度における）
DPI	dry powder inhaler	粉末製剤吸入器
DPTワクチン	diphtheria-pertussis-tetanus vaccine	三種（ジフテリア・百日咳・破傷風）混合ワクチン
DRG/PPS	diagnosis related group/prospective payment system	診断群別包括支払方式
DS	dry syrup	ドライシロップ
DSM	diagnostic and statistical manual of mental disorders	精神障害の診断と統計の手引き
DSU	Drug Safety Update	医薬品安全対策情報
DV	domestic violence	家庭内暴力（ドメスティック・バイオレンス）
DVT	deep vein thrombosis	深在静脈血栓症
DW	distilled water	蒸留水
Dx	diagnosis	診断

E

E-drug	essential drug	必須医薬品
E/N比	essential amino acids/non-essential amino acids ratio	必須アミノ酸/非必須アミノ酸比
EAA	essential amino acid	必須アミノ酸
EB	epidermal burn	Ⅰ度熱傷
EBM	evidence-based medicine	科学的根拠に基づく医療
EC	effective concentration	有効濃度
EC	emergency contraceptive	緊急避妊薬
EC/TC	esterified cholesterol to total cholesterol ratio	コレステロールエステル/総コレステロール比
EC_{50}	50% effective concentration	50%有効濃度
ECD	electrochemical detector	電気化学検出器

ECG	electrocardiogram	心電図
ED	elemental diet	成分栄養
ED_{50}	50% effective dose	50%有効量
EDA	exploratory data analysis	探索的データ解析
EDC	electronic data capture	電子データ収集
EEG	electroencephalogram	脳波
EF	ejection fraction	駆出率
EFA	essential fatty acid	必須脂肪酸
EGF	epidermal growth factor	上皮細胞増殖因子
eGFR	estimated glomerular filtration rate	推算糸球体濾過量
Eh	hepatic extraction	肝抽出率
EIA	environmental impact assessment	環境アセスメント（環境影響評価）
EIA	enzyme immunoassay	酵素免疫測定法
ELISA	enzyme-linked immunosorbent assay	エライザ法
ELISA	enzyme-linked immunosorbent assay	酵素結合免疫測定法
EM	extensive metabolizer	高代謝能保持者
EMG	electromyogram	筋電図
EMR	electronic medical record	電子診療録
EN	enteral nutrition	経腸栄養法
EPPV	early postmarketing phase vigilance	市販直後調査
ER	emergency room	救急治療室
ES cell	embryonic stem cell	ES 細胞，胚性幹細胞
ESR	electron spin resonance	電子スピン共鳴
ESR	erythrocyte sedimentation rate	赤血球沈降速度

F

Fab	antigen-binding fragment	抗原結合性フラグメント
FAPA	Federation of Asian Pharmaceutical Association	アジア薬剤師連盟
FAS	full analysis set	最大の解析対象集団
FBS	fasting blood sugar	空腹時血糖
FD	faculty development	大学教員資質開発
FDA	Food and Drug Administration	米国食品医薬品局
FEV_1	forced expiratory volume in 1 sec	呼吸1秒量
FF	filtration fraction	ろ過率
FFP	fresh frozen plasma	新鮮凍結血漿
FIC index	fractional inhibitory concentration index	薬理学的協力作用を表す指標
FIM	first-in-man (human) study	ヒト初回投与試験

FIP　International Pharmaceutical Federation　国際薬剤師・薬学連合
FOI　Freedom Of Information　情報開示
FPMAJ　The Federation of Pharmaceutical Manufacturers' Associations of Japan　日本製薬団体連合会
FT　Fourier transform　フーリエ変換
FTU　finger tip unit　塗布量の単位

G

GABA　γ-aminobutyric acid　γ-アミノ酪酸
GC-MS　gas chromatography-mass spectrometry　ガスクロマトグラフ質量分析
GCP　Good Clinical Practice　医薬品の臨床試験の実施の基準
GCT　glucose challenge test　ブドウ糖チャレンジ試験
GDP　Gross Domestic Production　国内総生産
GE　generic drug　後発医薬品，ジェネリック医薬品
GER　gastric emptying rate　胃排出速度
GET　gastric emtying time　胃内容排出時間
GFR　glomerular filtration rate　糸球体濾過速度
GI　gastrointestinal　胃腸の，消化管の
GILSP　Good Industrial Large Scale Practice　優良工業製造規範
GLP　Good Laboratory Practice　医薬品の安全性に関する非臨床試験の実施の基準
GLP-1　glucagon-like peptide-1　グルカゴン様ペプチド-1
GLUT　glucose transporter　グルコース輸送担体
GMP　Good Manufacturing Practice　医薬品及び医薬部外品の製造管理及び品質管理の基準
GNP　Gross National Product　国民総生産
GOT(AST)　glutamic oxaloacetic transaminase　グルタミン酸オキザロ酢酸トランスアミラーゼ
GP　general practitioner　一般開業医
GPEP　Good Pharmacy Education Practice　薬学教育に関する規範
GPP　Good Pharmacy Practice　薬局業務規範
GPSP　Good Postmarketing Study Practice　医薬品の製造販売後調査の実施の基準
GPT(ALT)　glutamic pyruvic transaminase　グルタミン酸ピルビン酸トランスアミナーゼ
GQP　Good Quality Practice　製造販売品質保証基準（製造販売後の品質管理の基準）
GSP　Good Supplying Practice　医薬品の供給と品質確保に関する実践規範
GTT　glucose tolerance test　耐糖能試験，ブドウ糖負荷試験
GVHD　graft versus host disease　移植片対宿主病

GVP Good Vigilance Practice 製造販売後安全管理の基準

H

HCC hepatocellular carcinoma 肝細胞がん
HCU high care unit 高度治療室
HDF hemodiafiltration 血液透析濾過
HEN home enteral nutrition 在宅経腸栄養
HEPA filter high efficiency particulate air filter ヘパフィルター(高性能エアフィルター)
HLA human leukocyte antigen ヒト白血球(型)抗原
HIS hospital information system 病院情報システム
HIV human immunodeficiency virus ヒト免疫不全ウイルス
HMG-CoA 3-hydroxy-3-methylglutaryl coenzyme A 3-ヒドロキシ-3-メチルグルタリル補酵素 A
HMO Health Maintenance Organization 米国健康維持機構
HOT 番号 HOT reference code ホット番号(標準医薬品マスターコード)
HPLC high performance liquid chromatography 高速液体クロマトグラフィー
HR hazard ratio ハザード比
HSCT hematopoietic stem cell transplantation 造血幹細胞移植

I

i.a. intraarterial injection (infusion) 動脈内注射
i.c. intracutaneous injection 皮内注射
i.d. intradermal injection 皮内注射
i.m. intramuscular injection 筋肉内注射
i.p. intraperitoneal injection 腹腔内注射
i.t. intrathecal injection 脊髄腔内注射
i.v. intravenous injection 静脈内注射
IAP international accreditation program 医療機能評価・認定の国際協調プログラム
IB investigator's brochure 治験薬概要書
IBW ideal body weight 標準体重
IC informed consent インフォームド・コンセント(医師等から説明を受けた上での説明と同意)
IC$_{50}$ 50% inhibitory concentration 50%阻害濃度
ICC in-country care-taker 治験国内管理人
ICC Infection Control Committee 感染制御委員会

ICD　infection control doctor　感染制御医師
ICD　International Statistical Classification of Diseases and Related Health Problems　国際疾病分類（疾病および関連保健問題の国際統計分類）
ICH　International Conference on Harmonization on Technical Requirements for Registration of Pharmaceuticals for Human Use　日米EU医薬品規制調和国際会議
ICT　infection control team　院内感染制御チーム
ICU　intensive care unit　集中治療室
IDDM　insulin dependent diabetes mellitus　1型糖尿病，インスリン依存性糖尿病
IDMC　independent data-monitoring committee　効果安全性評価委員会，独立データモニタリング委員会
IDT　intradermal test　皮内テスト
IEP　immunoelectrophoresis　免疫電気泳動法
IF　impact factor　インパクトファクター（科学雑誌の評価指標）
IF　interview form　インタビューフォーム
INDA　investigational new drug application　臨床試験実施申請資料
INN　international nonproprietary name　国際一般名称
iPS cell　induced pluripotent stem cell　人工多能性幹細胞
IRB　Institutional Review Board　臨床研究審査委員会
IS　internal standard　内部標準物質
ISA　intrinsic sympathomimetic activity　内因性交感神経刺激作用
ISO　International Organization for Standardization　国際標準化機構
ITT　intention to treat analysis　ITT解析

J

J-PEM　prescription-event monitoring in Japan　日本版処方イベントモニタリング
JAMS　The Japanese Association of Medical Sciences　日本医学会
JANコード　Japanese Article Number Code　流通コード
JAPIC　Japan Pharmaceutical Information Center　日本医薬情報センター
JCAHO　Joint Commission on Accreditation of Healthcare Organizations　医療施設認同認定機構（米国）
JCQHC　Japan Council for Quality Health Care　日本医療機能評価機構
JIS　Japanese Industrial Standard　日本工業規格
JMA　Japan Medical Association　日本医師会
JNA　Japanese Nursing Association　日本看護協会
JOP　JSPHCS Certified Oncology Pharmacist　日本医療薬学会がん専門薬剤師
JP　the Japanese Pharmacopeia　日本薬局方
JPA　Japan Pharmaceutical Association　日本薬剤師会

JPEC	Japan Pharmacists Education Center	日本薬剤師研修センター
JPMA	The Japan Pharmaceutical Manufacturers Association	日本製薬工業協会
JSHP	Japanese Society of Hospital Pharmacists	日本病院薬剤師会
JSOP	JSPHCS Certified Senior Oncology Pharmacist	日本医療薬学会がん指導薬剤師
JSPHCS	Japanese Society of Pharmaceutical Health Care and Sciences	日本医療薬学会

K

k_a	absorption rate constant	吸収速度定数
k_e	elimination rate constant	消失速度定数
k_i	inhibition constant	阻害定数
KJ	Kawakita Jiro method	KJ法
k_m	Michaelis constant	ミカエリス定数

L

LAN	local area network	構内通信網
LC/MS	liquid chromatography-mass spectrometry	液体クロマトグラフ質量分析計
LC/MS/MS	liquid chromatography-tandem mass spectrometry	液体クロマトグラフィー・タンデム質量分析法
LD	lethal dose	致死量
LD$_{100}$	100% lethal dose	確実致死量
LD$_{50}$	50% lethal dose	50％致死量
log PO/W	octanol/water partition coefficient	オクタノール・水分配係数
LS	learning strategy	学習方略

M

MARTA	multi-acting-receptor-targeted-antipsychotics	多元受容体標的化抗精神病薬
MBC	minimum bactericidal concentration	最小殺菌濃度
MCQ	multiple choice question	多肢選択問題
MD	medical doctor	医師
MDC	major diagnostic category	主要診断群（DPCのための疾患分類）
MDI	metered dose inhaler	噴霧式定量吸入器
MDR	multiple drug resistance	多剤耐性
ME	medical electronics	医用電子工学
MEC	minimum effective concentration	最小有効濃度
MED	minimum effective dose	最小有効量

MedDRA medical dictionary for regulatory activities　医薬規制用語集(ICH 国際医薬用語集)
MEDIS Medical Information System Development Center　医療情報システム開発センター
MEXT Ministry of Education, Culture, Sports, Science and Technology　文部科学省
MHC major histocompatibility gene complex　主要組織適合遺伝子複合体
MHLW Ministry of Health, Labour and Welfare　厚生労働省
MIC minimum inhibitory concentration　最小発育阻止濃度
MIC_{50} 50% minimum inhibitory concentration　50%最小発育阻止濃度
MIC_{90} 90% minimum inhibitory concentration　90%最小発育阻止濃度
MID minimum inhibitory dose　最小抑制量
miRNA micro RNA　マイクロ RNA
MLD minimum lethal dose　最小致死量
MMR measles-mumps-rubella vaccine　新三種混合ワクチン(麻疹，ムンプス，風疹)
MOA mechanism of action　作用機序
MOF multiple organ failure　多臓器不全
MPD maximum permissible dose　最大許容線量
MR medical representative　医薬情報担当者
MRI magnetic resonance imaging　核磁気共鳴画像法
MRP multidrug resistance related protein　多剤耐性関連タンパク質
MRT mean residence time　平均滞留時間
MS marketing specialist　医薬品卸販売担当者
MST median survival time　生存期間中央値
MSW medical sorcial worker　医療福祉相談員
MT medical technologist　臨床検査技師
MTC minimum toxic concentration　最小中毒濃度
MTD maximum tolerance dose　最大耐量
MVA multivariate analysis　多変量解析

N

n sample size　標本数
NAT nucleic acid amplification test　核酸増幅検査
NCQA National Committee for Quality Assurance　米国品質保証委員会
ncRNA non-coding RNA　機能性 RNA
ncRNA non-coding RNA　ノンコーディング RNA(非翻訳性 RNA)
NCU neurosurgical care unit　脳神経外科集中治療室
NDA new drug application　新薬の承認申請

NGO	Non-Governmental Organization	非政府組織
NHI	National Health Insurance	国民健康保険
NHS	national health service	国民保健サービス
NICE	National Institute for Health and Clinical Excellence	英国国立医療技術評価機構
NICU	neonatal intensive care unit	新生児集中治療部
NIDDM	non-insulin-dependent diabetes mellitus	2型糖尿病, インスリン非依存性糖尿病
NIH	National Institute of Health	米国国立衛生研究所
NIHS	National Institute of Health Sciences	国立医薬品食品衛生研究所
NMR	nuclear magnetic resonance	核磁気共鳴
NNH	number needed to harm	有害必要数
NNT	number needed to treat	治療必要数
NOAEL	no-observed-adverse-effect level	最大無有害量(無毒性量)
NOEL	no observed effect level	無影響量
NP	nurse practitioner	特定看護師(米)
NPO	Non-Profit Organization	特定非営利活動法人
NST	nutrition support team	栄養サポートチーム

O

O	objective data	客観的情報
O/W型	oil in water type	水中油型
OBME	outcome-based medical education	成果基盤型医学教育
OD	orphan drug	希少疾病用医薬品
ODA	Official Development Assistance	政府開発援助
ODP	one dose package	一包化
ODT	oral-disintegrating tablet	口腔内崩壊錠
Off-JT	off the job training	集合教育
OGTT	oral glucose tolerance test	経口糖負荷試験
OI	opportunistic infection	日和見感染症
OJT	on the job training	実地訓練(職場内教育)
OR	odds ratio	オッズ比
OS	overall survival time	全生存期間
OSCE	objective structured clinical examination	客観的臨床能力試験
Osm	osmolality(osmotic pressure)	浸透圧
OT	occupational therapist	作業療法士
OTC	over the counter drug	一般用医薬品

P

P p value P値(有意確率)
P-drug personal drug Pドラッグ(EBMに基づいてよく使う医薬品)
p.o. per os 経口投与
Pa$_{CO_2}$ arterial CO_2 pressure 動脈血二酸化炭素分圧
PAGE polyacrylamide gel electrophoresis ポリアクリルアミドゲル電気泳動
PAL Pharmaceutical Affairs Law 薬事法
Pa$_{O_2}$ arterial O_2 pressure 動脈血酸素分圧
PBL problem based learning 問題基盤型学習
PC partition coefficient 分配係数
PC pharmaceutical care 薬学的ケア
PCA patient controlled analgesia 自己調節鎮痛法
PCR polymerase chain reaction ポリメラーゼ連鎖反応
PCU palliative care unit 緩和ケア病棟
PD pharmacodynamics 薬力学
PD progressive disease 増悪(病状の進行)
PDCA plan do check action cycle(Deming's cycle) PDCAサイクル(デミングサイクル)
PDF portable document format ピーディーエフ
PE plasma exchange 血漿交換
PEG percutaneous endoscopic gastrostomy 経皮的内視鏡胃瘻造設術
PET positron emission tomography 陽電子放射断層撮影
PFS progression free survival 無増悪生存期間
PG Pharmacogenetics 薬理遺伝学
Pgp P-glycoprotein P-糖タンパク(MDR1)
PGx pharmacogenomics ファーマコゲノミクス
PH past history 既往歴
pI isoelectric point 等電点
PI present illness 現症
PK pharmacokinetics 薬物動態学
PK/PD pharmacokinetic/pharmacodynamic 薬物動態と薬力学
PL法 Product Liability Law PL法(製造物責任法)
PLM product life cycle management 製品のライフサイクルマネジメント(製品の販売推移)
PM poor metabolizer 低代謝能者
PMDA Pharmaceuticals and Medical Devices Agency 医薬品医療機器総合機構
PMDEC Pharmaceuticals and Medical Devices Evaluation Center 医薬品医療機器審査センター

PMS postmarketing surveillance 製造販売後調査（市販後調査）
PN parenteral nutrition 非経口栄養
POMR problem oriented medical record 問題指向型診療録
POS problem oriented system 問題指向型解決システム
PP per protocol analysis PP 解析
PPK population pharmacokinetics 母集団薬物動態
ppm parts per million (ex. 1mg/L = 1ppm) 100 万分の 1
PPN peripheral parenteral nutrition 末梢静脈栄養
PR partial response 部分奏効
PRTR pollutant release and transfer register 環境汚染物質排出移動登録
PS performance status 全身状態
PSJ The Pharmaceutical Society of Japan 日本薬学会
PT physical therapist 理学療法士
PT-INR prothrombin time-international normalized ratio プロトロンビン時間国際標準比
PTP press through package ピーティーピー包装
PTSD posttraumatic stress disorder 外傷後ストレス障害
PV pharmacovigilance 薬剤監視

Q

QA quality assurance 品質保証
QALY quality adjusted life year 生活の質を考慮した生存年
QAU quality assurance unit 信頼性保証部門（品質保証部門）
QC quality control 品質管理
QOL quality of life 生活の質（人生の質）
QR code quick response code QR コード（二次元バーコード）
QSAR quantitative structure-activity relationship 定量的構造活性相関

R

r correlation coefficient 相関係数
RCA root cause analysis 根本原因分析
RCT randomized controlled trial ランダム化比較試験
RD registered dietitian 管理栄養士
REE resting energy expenditure 安静時エネルギー消費量
REID reemerging infectious disease 再興感染症
REM 睡眠 rapid eye movement sleep レム睡眠

RFS	relapse-free survival	無再発生存期間
RIA	radioimmunoassay	ラジオイムノアッセイ(放射免疫測定)
RM	rapid metabolizer	迅速代謝能保持者
RP	role play	役割練習
RRR	relative risk reduction	相対リスク減少
RT-PCR	reverse transcriptase-polymerase chain reaction	逆転写酵素-ポリメラーゼ連鎖反応法
RTC	round-the-clock therapy	24時間維持療法

S

s.c.	subcutaneous injection	皮下注射
s.g.	specific gravity	比重
Sa$_{O_2}$	arterial O$_2$ saturation	動脈血酸素飽和度
SAR	structure-activity relationship	構造活性相関
SBA	summary basis of approval	新医薬品承認審査概要
SBOs	specific behavioral objectives	行動目標
SBR	summary basis of re-examination	新医薬品再審査概要
SBT	single-blind test	単盲検試験
SCJ	Science Council of Japan	日本学術会議
SCU	stroke care unit	脳卒中集中治療室
SD	stable disease	症状の安定
SD	standard deviation	標準偏差
SDV	source data(document) verification	原資料の直接閲覧による整合性確認
SEM	standard error of the mean	標準誤差
SGD	small group discussion	小グループ討論
SHELモデル	SHEL model	シェル・モデル
SM	safety margin	安全域
SMO	site management organization	治験施設支援機関
SNP(s)	single nucleotide polymorphism	一塩基多型
SOP	standard operating procedures	標準業務手順書
SP	simulated patient	模擬患者
SP	standard precautions	標準予防策
SPD	supply processing and distribution	外部業務委託
SPF	specific pathogen-free animal	SPF動物(特定の病原菌を持たない動物)
SP包装	strip package	ストリップ包装(ヒートシール包装の一種)
SQC	statistical quality control	統計的品質管理
SS	steady state	定常状態

SSM	simple suspension method	簡易懸濁法
STEM	scanning transmission electron microscope	走査透過型電子顕微鏡
STI	sexually transmitted infection	性感染症

T

T-Bil	total bilirubin	総ビリルビン
t$_{1/2}$	elimination half-life	消失半減期
TDM	therapeutic drug monitoring	治療薬物モニタリング
Tg	transgenic animal	トランスジェニック動物（形質転換動物）
TK	toxicokinetics	毒物動態学
TLO	technology licensing organization	技術移転機関
TLV	threshold limit values	暴露許容濃度
TLV-C	threshold limit values-ceiling value	天井値
T$_{max}$	time to maximum drug concentration	最高血中濃度到達時間
TNM 分類	tumor-nodes-metastasis classification	TNM 分類（国際対がん連合）
TPN	total parenteral nutrition	完全静脈栄養法
TTS	transdermal therapeutic system	経皮吸収型製剤
TWA	time weighted average	時間加重平均値

U

UDC	universal decimal classification	国際十進分類法
UICC	International Union against Cancer	国際対がん連合
UM	ultrarapid metabolizer	超迅速代謝能保持者
UMIN	University hospital Medical Information Network	大学病院医療情報ネットワーク
UNESCO	United Nations Educational, Scientific and Cultural Organization	ユネスコ（国連教育科学文化機関）
UNICEF	United Nations International Children's Emergency Fund	ユニセフ（国連国際児童緊急基金，国連児童基金）
USAN	United States Adopted Name	米国一般名
USI	urgent safety information	緊急安全性情報
USP	United States Pharmacopeia	米国薬局方

V

VAS	visual analog scale	視覚的アナログスケール

Vd   distribution volume   分布容積
V$_{max}$ maximum reaction velocity   最大反応速度

W

WAM   Welfare and Medical Service Agency   福祉医療機構
W/O 型   water in oil type   油中水型
WDS   withdrawal syndrome   退薬症候, 離脱症候群
WHO   World Health Organization   世界保健機関
WMA   World Medical Association   世界医師会
WS   workshop   ワークショップ

Y

YAM   young adult mean   若年成人平均値

付　録

○処 方 略 語
○アミノ酸略記

処方略語

略語	日本語	ラテン語	英語	ドイツ語
a.c.	食前	ante cibos	before meals	von dem Essen
aa.	各々	ana	of each	
ad	〜まで，全量	ad	to, up to	
ad lib.	適宜	ad libitum	at pleasure	
auf 1x tägl	1日1回	una in die	once a day	auf einmal täglich
auf 2x tägl	1日2回	bis in die	twice a day	auf zweimal täglich
auf 3x tägl	1日3回	ter in die	three times a day	auf dreimal täglich
auf 4x tägl	1日4回	qiater in die	four times a day	auf viermal täglich
auf 4x6 st""und	6時間毎に4回		4 times every 6 hours	aus 4xTage Sede 6 St""un
b.d.S.	授乳時		at breast feeding	bei der Stillung
b.i.d.	1日2回	bis in die	twice a day	auf zweimal täglich
b.s.	頓服	bei schmerz		
Cito!	至急	Cito!	quickly	
dieb.alt.	隔日	diebus alternis	every other day	
div.	分割せよ	divide	divide	
f., F.	調製せよ	fiat	make, let to be make	
ft.	調製せよ	fiat	make, let to be make	
G ( ) TD	〜日分投与		give ( ) days	tage Dosen
gtt.	滴	gutta, guttae	drop	
h.febr.	発熱時	hora febre	at pyrexia	beim Pyrexie
h.s.	就寝前	hora somni	at bedtime	von dem Schlafengehen
hor.una.a.c.	食前1時間	hora una ante cibos	one hour before meals	
hor.una.p.c.	食後1時間	hora una post cibos	one hour after meals	
i.c.	食間	inter cibos	between meals	zwischen dem Essen
m.	朝	mane	morning	morgens
M.&A.	朝・夕		morning and evening	Morgen und Abend
M.m.	混和せよ	misce	mixture	

略語	日本語	ラテン語	英語	ドイツ語
mer.d	昼	merdie	noon	mittag
n.	夜	noctis	night	nacht
n.d.E	食後	post cibos	after meals	nach dem Essen
O.D.	右眼	Oculo Dextro	right eye	
O.L.	左眼	Oculo Laevo, Oculo Sinnistro	left eye	
O.S.	左眼	Oculo Laevo, Oculo Sinnistro	left eye	
O.U.	両眼	Oculo Uterque	each eye	
ODP	一包化		one dose package	
omn.man	毎朝	omni mane	every morning	
omn.noct.	毎夜	omni nocte	every night	
p.c.	食後	post cibos	after meals	nach dem Essen
p.r.n.	必要時	pro re nate	when necessary	
q.3h.	3時間毎	quaque 3 hora	every three hours	mit jedem 3 Stunde
q.d.	毎日	quaque die	every day (daily)	jeden Tag
q.i.d.	1日4回	qiater in die	four times a day	auf viermal täglich
q.s.	適量	quantum suffcit	as much as sufficient	
q4.h.	4時間毎	quaque 4 hora	every four hours	mit jedem 4 Stunde
S.	用法	Signa	direction for use	
sofort n.d.E.	食直後	statim post cibos	immediately after meals	sofort nach dem Essen
stat.	直ちに	statium	immediately	
stat.p.c.	食直後	statim post cibos	immediately after meals	sofort nach dem Essen
sum.	服用せよ	sumenda	to be taken	
t.i.d.	1日3回	ter in die	three times a day	auf dreimal täglich
u.d.	用法口授	ut dictum	as directed	
u.i.d.	1日1回	una in die	once a day	auf einmal täglich
ut dict	用法口授	ut dictum	as directed	
v.	夕	vespere	evening	abend s
v.d.E	食前	ante cibos	before meals	von dem Essen

略語	日本語	ラテン語	英語	ドイツ語
v.d.S	就寝前	hora somni	at bedtime	von dem Schlafengehen
z.d.E	食間	inter cibos	between meals	zwischen dem Essen

アミノ酸略記

1文字表記	3文字表記	名称
A	Ala	Alanine　アラニン
B	Asx	アスパラギン酸またはアスパラギン
C	Cys	Cysteine　システイン
D	Asp	Aspartic acid　アスパラギン酸
E	Glu	Glutamic acid　グルタミン酸
F	Phe	Phenylalanine　フェニルアラニン
G	Gly	Glycine　グリシン
H	His	Histidine　ヒスチジン
I	Ile	Isoleucine　イソロイシン
K	Lys	Lysine　リシン
L	Leu	Leucine　ロイシン
M	Met	Methionine　メチオニン
N	Asn	Asparagine　アスパラギン
P	Pro	Proline　プロリン
Q	Gln	Glutamine　グルタミン
R	Arg	Arginine　アルギニン
S	Ser	Serine　セリン
T	Thr	Threonine　スレオニン
U	Sec	Selenocysteine　セレノシステイン
V	Val	Valine　バリン
W	Trp	Tryptophan　トリプトファン
X	Xaa	未知またはその他のアミノ酸
Y	Tyr	Tyrosine　チロシン
Z	Glx	グルタミン酸またはグルタミン

参考図書等一覧

【参考図書】

医薬実務用語集 第 12 版　薬事日報社・編著（薬事日報社）1999 年
医療安全用語事典　日本病院管理学会・著（エルゼビア・ジャパン）2004 年
医療の質用語事典　棟近雅彦，飯田修平，飯塚 悦・監（日本規格協会）2005 年
医療・病院管理用語事典 改訂第 3 版　日本病院管理学会学術情報委員会・編（エルゼビア・ジャパン）2006 年
医療・病院管理用語事典 新版　日本医療・病院管理学会学術情報委員会（市ヶ谷出版社）2011 年
化学物質環境・安全管理用語事典 改訂第 3 版　環境・安全管理用語編集委員会・編（化学工業日報社）2005 年
最新医学大辞典 第 2 版　最新医学大辞典編集委員会・編（医歯薬出版）1996 年
調剤学総論 改訂第 10 版　堀岡正義・著（南山堂）2011 年
南山堂医学大辞典 第 19 版（南山堂）2006 年
日常診療に役立つ抗感染症薬の PK-PD　戸塚恭一，三鴨廣繁・監（ユニオンエース）2010 年
日本環境感染学会用語集　日本環境感染学会用語委員会（日本環境感染学会）2010
病院感染用語辞典　木村 哲，大久保憲，岸下雅通，広瀬千也子・編（医薬ジャーナル社）2000 年
薬学用語辞典　日本薬学会・編（東京化学同人）2012 年
薬剤師のための感染制御マニュアル 第 3 版　日本病院薬剤師会・監（薬事日報社）2012 年
臨床薬理学用語集 第 2 版　日本臨床薬理学会用語編集委員会・編（ライフサイエンス出版）2009 年
臨床薬理学 第 2 版　日本臨床薬理学会（医学書院）2003 年

【参考ウェブページ】

医薬業界用語集　日本製薬工業協会（http://www.jpma.or.jp/glossary/）
治験ナビ用語集　治験ナビ（http://www.chikennavi.net/i_word_index.htm）
日本 TDM 学会専門用語解説　日本 TDM 学会（http://jstdm.umin.jp/yogo/yogo.html）
日本薬局方対訳集　MCL（http://www.mcl-corp.jp/software/t_phamacopeia.html）
薬学用語解説　日本薬学会（http://www.pharm.or.jp/dictionary/wiki.cgi）

医療薬学用語集

定価　本体2,700円（税別）

平成26年3月25日　発　行

編　集	一般社団法人 日本医療薬学会 用語集編集委員会
発行人	武田　正一郎
発行所	株式会社　じほう

　　　　101-8421　東京都千代田区猿楽町1-5-15（猿楽町SSビル）
　　　　電話　編集　03-3233-6361　販売　03-3233-6333
　　　　振替　00190-0-900481
　　　＜大阪支局＞
　　　　541-0044　大阪市中央区伏見町2-1-1（三井住友銀行高麗橋ビル）
　　　　電話　06-6231-7061

©2014　　　　　　　　　　　　　組版・印刷　㈱日本制作センター
Printed in Japan

本書の複写にかかる複製，上映，譲渡，公衆送信（送信可能化を含む）の各権利は株式会社じほうが管理の委託を受けています。

|JCOPY|＜(社)出版者著作権管理機構　委託出版物＞
本書の無断複写は著作権法上での例外を除き禁じられています。
複写される場合は，そのつど事前に，(社)出版者著作権管理機構（電話 03-3513-6969，FAX 03-3513-6979，e-mail：info@jcopy.or.jp）の許諾を得てください。

万一落丁，乱丁の場合は，お取替えいたします。
ISBN 978-4-8407-4576-5